"I hope that this doesn't sound hysterical to you, but I've gone on for five years thinking that I am just abnormal, and reading your book, I know I'm not."

BEVERLY S.

"Dr. Rako, I cannot thank you enough for all the work you have done in researching this great book. Since I am in the medical field, I know there are no guarantees, but your book has given me something I had not had in almost three years: validation and hope."

MARY ANN L.

"Since I bgan the testosterone six weeks ago, I want to tell you I am great! I am really great! I have never been better."

JANICE R.

"The reality of many women's plight exists—far more frequently than anyone realizes or admits. WHO WOULD BELIEVE THAT, IN 1999, THIS IGNORANCE EXISTS?" Thank you, Dr. Rako, for paving the way and opening closed doors."

CARLA B.

"Dr. Rako, after seeing you on TV and reading your book, I just put my head down on the table and cried. All the things I recognized in the book, I have experienced for the past seventeen years, since my hysterectomy. I really do wonder why my very attractive husband has even stayed with me."

DIANE M.

"I have felt very defeated regarding my doctor, who thinks I'm crazy, thinks it's in my mind, but I have no sexual desire. I'm in tears, but they are happy tears, because I think there's hope now."

SUZANNE G.

"I just am writing to tell you that I had seen you on the *Today* show, read your book and am now using topical testosterone, and I can't thank you enough. You have just changed my life . . ."

BARBARA T.

The Hormone *of* Desire

THE TRUTH ABOUT
TESTOSTERONE,
SEXUALITY, *and*
MENOPAUSE

Susan Rako, M.D.

Three Rivers Press   NEW YORK

*The information in this book is educational in nature
and is not intended to substitute for or to supersede
individual responsible medical consultation.*

Published by Three Rivers Press, New York, New York.
Member of the Crown Publishing Group.

Originally published in hardcover by Harmony Books, January 1996.
First paperback edition printed in 1999.

Random House, Inc. New York, Toronto, London, Sydney, Auckland
www.randomhouse.com

THREE RIVERS PRESS is a registered trademark and
the Three Rivers Press colophon is a trademark of Random House, Inc.

Printed in the United States of America

Library of Congress Cataloging-in-Publication Data
Rako, Susan.
The hormone of desire : the truth about testosterone, sexuality, and
menopause / by Susan Rako.
    Includes index.
    1. Menopause-Hormone therapy. 2. Testosterone-Therapeutic use.
3. Middle-aged women-Sexual behavior. 4. Testosterone-Physiological
effect. I. Title
RG186.R345 1995
612.6—dc20   95-174598
                    CIP

ISBN 0-609-80386-7

10 9 8 7 6 5 4 3

I dedicate this book to my daughter,
Jennifer Sarah Rako Bernardo,
whose love
and particular qualities of character and beauty
reflect, inspire, and support my best efforts.
And to her daughter,
Alexandra Grace

❧ Acknowledgments ❧

I can testify to the truth of Goethe's observation that "the moment one definitely commits oneself, then providence moves too. All sorts of things occur to help one that would never otherwise have occurred."

My gratitude for the providential assistance, generosity of spirit, patience, and wisdom of Ruth Hapgood, Sandra Goroff-Mailly, Jennifer Rako, Thomas Bernardo, Ed Klaiber, Manya Arond, John Taylor, Jeanne Mayell, and Sandra Lotz Fisher.

Catalytic contributors to this effort include Ted Kaptchuck, Deborah Rose, Daniel Federman, Helen Singer Kaplan, Barbara Sherwin, Karen Manning, Sandra Forman, and Sue McGovern.

I have been blessed with the love and wisdom in support of this project of Elissa and Daniel Arons, Irwin Avery, Daniel Crown, Linda and Jay Land, Marie Harburger, Jo-Anne Dillman, Ezila do Canto, Allen Scheier, and Linda and Don Berman.

I wish to thank the women who offered the use of details of their lives and excerpts of their written communications as clinical examples and with generous intention that their experiences might be of help to others.

I appreciate my dad, Robert Mandell, for his unconditional love, prayers, and zest for life.

I appreciate my editor, Shaye Areheart, for her belief in this book and for her respect for the integrity of my writing.

As I complete a final edit of this manuscript, I hear again and again in my mind's ear the melody and words of a song I accompanied on the piano for Worcester Classical High's chorus. Apologies to the poet, W. E. Henley, for the one word I changed unconsciously to be more acceptable to me consciously. Set to stirring music, with a rhythmic opening by the basses, the initial verse of "Invictus" concludes with this, which I find to be my ultimate gratitude:

I thank whatever gods may be for my unalterable soul.

❧ Contents ❧

CONTENTS

*Indeed, Medicine claims always to make experience
the test of its procedures. Plato therefore was right
in saying that to become a true doctor, a man must
have experienced all the illnesses he means to cure
and all the accidents and circumstances on which he is
to give an opinion. . . . Truly I would trust such a man.
For the others guide us like the man who paints seas, reefs
and harbors while seated at his table and sails the model of
a ship there in all safety. Toss him into reality and he does
not know where to begin.*

Montaigne, *Essays*, bk. I [1580], ch. 13,
Of Experience

❧ Introduction ❧

Today, women of all ages have come to appreciate their potential for a fulfilling and enduring sexual life. Dr. Susan Rako has researched and written a landmark book. With the publication of *The Hormone of Desire,* we finally have detailed, complete, responsible information about testosterone deficiency and supplementation. Addressed to women and to their doctors, this book redefines the concept of hormone replacement therapy to include testosterone for the large population of women who need it for the maintenance of vital and sexual energy—whether their testosterone deficiency has been caused by natural aging and menopause, surgical removal of the ovaries, or the effects of chemotherapy.

To understand why this is such an important book, it is worth remembering that not long ago, women's sexuality was a subject cloaked in mystery, about which little scientific information was known. Sexual responsivity was thought to be a one-step process, beginning with lust and ending with orgasm. In keeping with this point of view, there was only one female sexual disorder—frigidity.

In their best-selling book, *Human Sexual Inadequacy,* published in 1970, Masters and Johnson described in meticulous detail the physiology of the sexual response cycle and popularized the concept that orgasm, in both sexes, is triggered by the same physiological mechanism. *The New Sex Therapy* (Kaplan, 1974) separated the excitement from the orgasm phase disorders in women, as had been previously done for men. This represented a breakthrough in treatment methodology, as did the *Disorders of Sexual Desire* (Kaplan, 1979), which introduced the concept of the desire phase of the cycle for both women and men. Theoretically, sexual dysfunction may arise from disruption of any of the three phases of the sexual response cycle—desire, arousal, or orgasm. In our patients with testosterone deficiency, we have observed disruption in all three.

The medical community has been slow to accept and incorporate testosterone replacement for women suffering from deficiency despite evidence in the medical literature of the last forty years that it can be helpful. This is not an uncommon occurrence. Research and treatment of female sexual dysfunction, particularly in older women, has traditionally received seriously little attention and funding, compared with allocations focused on male sexual dysfunction.

From our point of view as sexologists, for a woman to live with inadequate levels of testosterone is no small matter. For many it means the complete inability to experience sexual desire, sexual fantasy, arousal, and/or orgasm. The fact is that female sexuality without testosterone is a house without a foundation. No matter how hard a woman might try to assemble the building blocks of healthy sexual functioning—the required amounts of other hormones, a loving partner, adequate stimulation, possibly a good sexual fantasy—it cannot work if she does not have the basic foundation of enough testosterone. We have found that replacing the missing testosterone can restore a woman to her baseline level of sexual functioning.

We anticipate that *The Hormone of Desire* will create a groundswell of interest, to the point of inspiring many more physicians to learn what they need to know about testosterone deficiency and supplementation for women. We are delighted that both women who want to learn how to take care of themselves and health care professionals who treat them can turn to this meticulously researched book, annotated and documented with the body of core information on testosterone, as a guide and a resource.

Gracefully, intelligently, and sensitively written, *The Hormone of Desire* began as Dr. Rako's own story, a story of challenge, inspiration, and determination, and came to completion as a book that can benefit the millions of women who need testosterone replacement therapy for health and a better quality of life.

We applaud Dr. Rako for her groundbreaking work.

Barbara Bartlik, M.D.
Assistant Clinical Professor,
Department of Psychiatry
The New York Hospital—Cornell
University Medical College;
Staff, Human Sexuality Program,
Payne Whitney Psychiatric Clinic;
Past President, Women's Medical
Association of New York City

Helen Singer Kaplan, M.D., Ph.D.,
Clinical Professor, Department of Psychiatry
The New York Hospital—Cornell University
Medical College;
Director and Founder,
Human Sexuality Program,
Payne Whitney Psychiatric Clinic

↶ Foreword ↷

One Sunday, after a long day and night at Harvard's Countway Library lugging heavy medical journals from the stacks to the copying machines, glad to have located the articles I had hoped to find, I treated myself to an Indian dinner, pored over the copies I had made, called it a night, and had the following dream:

I am on a beach, near an expanse of ocean. Digging in the sand, I unearth many large seashells. Conches. Substantial, they seem beautiful to me, even though they are imperfect. It is apparent that someone else had found them in the ocean and discarded them on the beach, where, for some time, they have been covered with sand.

Digging farther, I discover a kind of grotto. I am aware that I must watch my footing, although the risk of falling does not appear to be great. The grotto is not very deep. One could not fall too far. And I find, also, the preserved carcass of a large fish, in its own way beautiful.

A story from my psyche, the dream speaks to me. The shells seem to be symbols for the old medical journal articles I have been "digging up"—material that is valuable to me today, although it has been buried in the archives, some of it, for decades. I think particularly of one paper by Dr. Sheldon

Waxenberg and his colleagues at the Sloan-Kettering Institute in New York and published in 1959.

An elegantly written paper, it is notably compassionate as well. The authors made use of their clinical observations of women with advanced breast cancer whose ovaries and adrenal glands had been removed in the hope of slowing progress of the disease. The study came to a conclusion that androgens, rather than estrogens, are responsible for sexual desire in the human female.

Potentially groundbreaking material. Imperfect, to be sure. One could pick it apart in many ways. But there is some strong truth here. We have to watch our footing, how we use all this.

And in the dream, that ossifying fish—primordial symbol of aging, substantial and beautiful even in its remains—transforming to endure, fossilize, yet to be known in some way?

As I write this, I remember my first reading of that paper from Sloan-Kettering. Along with the excitement I felt at reading their postulate of androgens as the hormones of desire, I felt some dizzying, long-buried pain.

The details of that study brought back the memory of a beloved aunt, my aunt Bess, who died of breast cancer in 1965, while I was still in medical school. During the long course of her illness, and when chemotherapy and radiation had failed, she consulted specialists at Sloan-Kettering. Maybe even these same doctors. In hopes of buying time, she accepted the radical choice of treatment that required her to have her ovaries and her adrenal glands removed.

She loved life, lived and died with courage and grace. Perhaps her extraordinary fight for life contributed to something lasting—knowledge now used to revitalize those of us living without mortal disease, fundamentally healthy, but deficient in a hormone, dead to our sexuality, lacking in vital energy and the feeling of vigorous well-being.

I will always remember my first day of medical school. September, 1962. The entering class convenes in the auditorium. The dean speaks.

"Primum non nocere."
"Above all, do no harm."
May the material in this book
be used only for the good of humankind.

The New York Times
Thursday, May 12, 1994

Low Testosterone
Affects Women, Too

To the Editor:

I have researched the medical literature and communicated with leading researchers in "female androgen deficiency syndrome" (testosterone deficiency), and conducted workshops to educate women suffering from a decrease in the normal, essential levels of this hormone. "Male Hormone Molds Women, Too, in Mind and Body" (Science Times, May 3) recognizes resistance to acknowledging the role of the "so-called male hormone" in women, and then extensively discusses *excess* testosterone.

It is more comfortable to consider treating women with too much "male hormone" than to look at the compromised quality of life for millions of women who have testosterone deficiency because of menopause or the too-often unnecessary removal of ovaries with hysterectomy or the chemically induced menopause following chemotherapy for cancer. Your article has a large illustration and forbidding list of "Effects of Excess of

Male Hormones," but none for the effects of testosterone deficiency. They would include loss of sexual desire, loss of sensation in clitoris and nipples, difficulty in reaching orgasm, thinning and loss of pubic hair, loss of vital energy and diminished sense of well-being, reduction in muscle tone, dulling and brittleness of scalp hair, skin dryness and, for some, atrophy of genital tissue not responsive to estrogen.

No woman considers the prospect of using supplementary testosterone without concern about potential side effects. But restoring a normal-range level of testosterone to a woman with deficiency cannot cause the effects you show accompanying testosterone excess.

Susan Rako, M.D.
Newtonville, Mass., May 3, 1994

1

HOW THIS BOOK

CAME TO BE

The material in this book represents the distillate of what I have learned in my research, in my own experience with testosterone and menopause, and in the feedback I have received from the hundreds of women who have consulted with me to learn about testosterone and to brainstorm about approaches to their symptoms of testosterone deficiency.

My experience began like that of many women approaching menopause. Always having been comfortable with my body's female manifestations and rhythms, I had expected to "go through menopause naturally"—without the use of hormones.

Twelve years ago, when I was forty-seven, still having menstrual periods—albeit irregularly—and several years *before* the eventuation of my menopause, I could not make sense of the significant loss in general vital energy, thinning and loss of pubic hair, and loss of sexual energy I experienced. To say that I was lacking a feeling of well-being would be an understatement.

Because I had a medical education, an early interest in reproductive endocrinology (and a character formed with a will to get to the bottom of things I cared about), I was not inclined to settle for the temporizing, patronizing, dismissive, and irresponsibly uninformed treatment I received from the gynecologists and endocrinologists I consulted. When my state of misery developed, I assumed that estrogen was what I needed, and resigned myself to the prospect of taking estrogen and progestin, but my conservative gynecologist was unwilling to prescribe estrogen until I had stopped having periods. I waited, feeling flatter and flatter, seeking out alternative methods to try to pick up my energies and revitalize my turned-off body.

I will never forget the humiliation I experienced in consultation with a well-respected male endocrinologist. I wanted his help in the matter of beginning estrogen therapy before menopause. I described my sexual deadness as carefully and completely as I could. Since libido is such a complex phenomenon in relationships, I wanted him to know that I had simple ways of knowing how dead, sexually, I was: My relationship with myself had been pretty dependable since I was a girl.

The doctor said, impatiently, "I can't possibly justify recommending hormones because you want to *masturbate.*" If a man had consulted this endocrinologist with the complaint that he had been accustomed to enjoying his libido, both with and without a partner, and was suffering sexual deadness, could he possibly have received such a response?

I am a physician, a psychiatrist, and a woman. I was embarrassed, and then angry—for myself and for all of us who struggle to get the help we need in matters we would prefer to keep private. And I knew that I would not quit until I was satisfied that I had done what I could to take care of myself. That was one of the reasons I had gone to medical school in the first place.

In a search to learn what I could find about loss of sexual and vital energy at menopause, I became very familiar with the stacks of Harvard's Countway Medical Library and of several other libraries.

The data was there.
But it didn't say estrogen was what I needed.
It said testosterone.

I found papers in the archives developing a substantial body of knowledge about the functions of testosterone for women, beginning with the 1940s publications by the late Dr. Robert Greenblatt, former professor of endocrinology at the Medical College of Georgia, who pioneered the use of testosterone for women. Among the several hundred relevant articles and books, I also found that groundbreaking paper published in 1959 by Dr. Waxenberg and his associates at New York's Sloan-Kettering Institute, offering evidence that *testosterone is the hormone responsible for the experience of sexual desire not only for men but also for women.*

I soon learned that research has shown:

1. A woman's normal physiology includes the production of a critical amount of testosterone, essential to her normal sexual development, to the healthy functioning of virtually all tissues in her body, and to her experience of vital energy and sexual libido.
2. This critical amount of testosterone decreases after menopause, in many women resulting in a loss of vital energy and sexual libido.
3. Supplementary testosterone can be a substantial help in restoring a woman to her familiar level of energy, libido, and well-being.
4. Only the use of irresponsibly high doses of testosterone over a sustained period of time can produce undesirable effects.

While I collected this compelling information, I continued to investigate and to try alternative approaches—herbs, acupuncture, homeopathy, massage. And I shopped around and found a gynecologist knowledgeable and experienced in prescribing estrogen and progestin for women before menopause. She did an endometrial biopsy, which is an office procedure whereby a small amount of tissue is removed from the lining of the uterus in order to check for possible signs of abnormal cells prior to the estrogen therapy. Upon finding the tissue normal, she prescribed estrogen and progestin, warning me to watch for and to report any "abnormal bleeding"—any bleeding from the vagina other than the bleeding expected after the progestin part of the cycle.

For the first few weeks, I felt some stimulation of energy, but after a month, I felt, if anything, "deader" than ever. Until I researched it for myself, I had no idea that this further loss of sexual libido was due to an effect of the supplemental estrogen—which makes *less available* whatever testosterone a woman may have.

My research taught me enough about the substantial reasons to take "traditional" hormone-replacement therapy—estrogen and progestin—that I made a clear decision to continue to do so. Finally, after a year and a half of using estrogen and progestin and learning about testosterone, I decided that a conservative course of supplemental testosterone was worth a try. Today—in July of 1998—in Boston, there are a few gynecologists who have some experience prescribing testosterone for women with symptoms of deficiency, but most still do not. Many are resistant to considering prescribing testosterone for women in *any* case. In 1987, I had a hard time finding one who would.

In my research, I had read of several methods of using testosterone. While menopause clinics in England and other countries use pellets that can be planted under the skin, testosterone pellets are not readily available in the United States. "Implants" did not appeal to me, in any event. Some physicians in Canada and in the United States, as well as in other parts of the world, prescribe monthly depot injections of testosterone. A "depot" is a suspension of any substance in an oil base, which is injected into muscle and tends to disperse into the general blood circulation gradually, over a period of time.

Not knowing how my body might react to testosterone, and aware that I might choose to stop treatment, I wanted to have control over how much hormone I was getting and how long the effects might last. Neither pellets nor depot injections could allow for this. The clinching factor for me in rejecting these methods was the research data that showed that women receiving depot injections or implants developed blood levels of testosterone much higher than the normal range. And I was discouraged to find that the testosterone available in pill form came in dosages higher than I was comfortable taking.

I had read of a method (described by Greenblatt) of applying a preparation of testosterone powder mixed with petroleum jelly in very small amounts directly to the genital tissue. Since my tissue appeared not to have benefited to a full degree from the estrogen I had been taking, it made sense to me (and to the woman who was now my fifth gynecologist) that I try using testosterone directly on the tissue.

The topical preparation did improve the tissue locally and was also absorbed into my general circulation. Within two months, and after five years, I felt "like myself again."

That was the beginning.

I realized that I had learned something that might help other women. In an attempt to share this information, I offered a workshop at a center for "education of mind and body" in Cambridge, Massachusetts. On a hot July evening in 1993, I gave my first talk to a packed room of women who came to learn about "sexual energy and menopause." I taught them and they reinforced for me what I had learned in ten years of exploring the phenomenon of menopause:

There can be as many differences in the experience of menopause, vital energy, and sexual energy from woman to woman as there are menopausal women.

A woman "sailing through menopause" is enjoying a constitutional balance not common to all women. A woman developing symptoms of testosterone deficiency in the years *before* menopause is suffering a constitutional balance not common to all women.

In my research, I've come to understand that a complex of factors contribute to the variety of experiences of menopause that different women have. For example, physiologic developments specific to the shutdown of the ovaries and the effects of this shutdown on the adrenal glands, together with factors of aging (on testosterone receptors, on enzyme functions, and on the adrenals), all contribute to the menopause experience, making it unique to each woman.

The popular metaphor for a hoped-for experience, "sailing through menopause," invites extension.

Menopause is a journey through poorly charted waters.

And some physicians approach the possibility of prescribing supplementary testosterone for women suffering symptoms of its deficiency with the resistance and ignorance of the sailors who believed that the earth was flat, and that if they proceeded to sail on, they would fall off.

In May 1994, the *New York Times* published an article on testosterone deficiency that was irresponsibly slanted. It acknowledged the phenomenon of testosterone deficiency, but focused primarily on the need to seek out and treat women with conditions of testosterone *excess*. How disheartening this is! I was taught about the pathological conditions of testosterone excess when I went to medical school in 1962. **The important news for women and their doctors in 1999 is the**

fact that conditions of testosterone deficiency do exist, need attention, and can be treated. That is something I didn't learn in medical school. And I would be surprised if it is regularly being taught today.

Focusing on this limiting bias, I wrote a letter to the *New York Times*, which they published on May 12, 1994, and is reprinted in full on page 21 of this book. As I complete this manuscript, I am still receiving telephone calls and letters from women all over the United States (certainly a testament to the widespread readership of the *New York Times*). The fact that so many women continue to write and call wanting to tell me their stories and asking for information tells me something about how hard it is for them to ask for and to get the help they need for symptoms of testosterone deficiency.

The following letter moved me particularly:

Dear Dr. Rako,

I am a woman fifty-two years of age and have been in menopause for a couple of years now. I initially tried to handle it "naturally," but after talking to several doctors I decided that perhaps it would be a good idea, after all, to use estrogen. I have had my uterus removed and therefore was a good candidate for the "patch." I was led to believe that it would help in protecting my bones from osteoporosis, my heart, and to keep my cholesterol levels in check.

In the past two to three years I have explained to four different gynecologists that since I have been in menopause I have experienced a loss of desire for sex, loss of pubic hair and some scalp hair, and a general sense of depression (something I have never been bothered by before). I have also started seeing a therapist to deal with some of the issues around depression and there certainly are environmental, situational, physical, and psychological reasons why I

29

could be feeling depressed and therefore not have much desire for sex.

Several weeks ago I saw your letter to the editor in the New York Times. I was so interested in what you had to say that I showed it to my health-care practitioner and to my therapist in the hopes that they would validate some of what you said. Instead the therapist kind of shrugged her shoulders, not knowing much about the problem, and suggested Prozac to me. The nurse practitioner I see at [a West Coast HMO] did not feel qualified to talk about it and suggested that I give a little more time to the use of the [estrogen] that I started on about a month ago and to also consider an antidepressant.

I feel like antidepressants are being pushed on me before trying treatment with something like testosterone, which may actually be what I need. I'm not a doctor and certainly don't know. I do know that I don't want to start taking antidepressants. I feel like the professionals don't know what else to do when someone complains about depression and loss of sex drive, so the first thing they do is to prescribe antidepressants.

I hope you won't consider this an invasion of your privacy. You included your name and your city in the paper and I was able to get the address from information. I just don't know who else to turn to for information or how to go about searching for good information on the use of testosterone for what is going on with my body and mind.

I would appreciate any information you might be willing to pass on.

This book is for you.
And for your doctors.

2

POORLY CHARTED WATERS

Since you are reading this book, you already know part of the problem. You have likely met up with the ignorance (within the medical community as well as the general population), fear, ideological resistance, and sexual politics (both feminist and chauvinist) that confound the treatment of women suffering from testosterone deficiency. A large part of our resistance to recognizing the phenomenon of testosterone deficiency in women may be our resistance to accepting that losses of energy and of sexual functioning can be a consequence of menopause and aging, when we expect still to be vigorous. Who wants to think about the possibility of losing the capacity for sexual desire as part of menopause?

If we are healthy, we expect to be energetic and sexually alive in our late thirties, forties, fifties—and the popular myth is that we *can*. But while some of us (with the genes for it) can, too many of us *cannot*.

First a word about libido—*women's* libido. In spite of the women's liberation movement, the sexual revolution, and the apparent implications of several popular books of women's sexual fantasies, many women are not comfortable recognizing sexual excitement if they don't have a partner. I found a number of women who responded to a question about the state of their libido with some version of "Libido? How should

I know? I don't have a man in my life." Native-American Seneca wisdom claims that "the man is the spark that lights the woman." A romantic, even a poetic statement—and true for the romantic poet in us (at least some of the time). But many of us know our rhythms of desire and know that these rhythms are, in some way, hormonal. And not necessarily dependent on the presence of an available partner. As one fifty-three-year-old woman said, "It has been a year since I had a partner, so I'm not sure how sex would be now, but I notice that I rarely have sexual fantasies anymore. I feel less 'alive' than I used to, and I don't like it."

Only five of the hundreds of research papers I read included any mention of sexual dreams, sexual fantasy, and masturbation as being relevant in evaluating the effects of hormones on women's sexual functioning. When I had the occasion to ask one research scientist about such an omission in a particular study, I learned that, initially, the women *were* asked how often they masturbated. About to undergo hysterectomy for various gynecological problems (not including malignancy), some women answered, "I'm about to have major surgery, and you are asking me about *that?*" Most studies of women where surgery was not an element at all still failed to inquire about "that."

"That" does seem to be a difficult subject, even for someone as notoriously liberated as Germaine Greer. From Greer's book on menopause, *The Change,* the following paragraph makes sense only if we read it as a reflection of Greer's personal sensibilities, inhibitions, and fantasies. In the world according to Greer:

> The administration of testosterone will bring about an instant increase in genital sensitivity, but the patient is very aware that this is unrelated to sexual response as she knows it. If a peri-menopausal woman is not part of a heterosexual couple, she will not be offered this treatment, for the diffuse genital tension she will feel

can only lead into dangerous and compromising situations or humiliating bouts of masturbation [my emphasis].

Egad. The peculiar concern about the "humiliation" of potential masturbation aside, whatever one might wish or fear, testosterone is no such aphrodisiac. If the administration of testosterone *could* bring about "an instant increase in genital sensitivity," there would probably be a pretty active street market for the drug. The common experience for women suffering testosterone deficiency is that it takes several weeks of carefully adjusted supplement to produce improvement in vital and sexual energy and sensation.

Greer's point about the heterosexual bias in the medical establishment does bear out. None of the women in any study of testosterone and sexuality reported in major medical journals was acknowledged to be homosexual. The research papers measured female sexual activity only in terms of intercourse. Moreover, women without a male partner were actually dropped from most studies. In the popular press, ignorance abounds. Browsing through the Dartmouth Bookstore recently, I found a book titled *How to Make Love to Your Aging Man,* which contained detailed information as to the kind of stimulation, the patience, the understanding an aging man needs. Any books addressed to the needs of aging women?

Instead, we encounter the "use it or lose it" school of female sexuality. This dumb approach claims that, if a woman has a functioning sexual partner, she is all set to keep herself functioning sexually well into old age. No mention about her appetite for sexual experience; no mention about her libido at all. Just the implication that, if she keeps her equipment in regular use, she'll be all set for sex until she crumps out altogether.

For a majority of women, without the use of supplementary estrogen, genital atrophy will eventually make the mechanics of sexual intercourse impossible. For too many women, without the use of supplementary testosterone, "libido atrophy" will significantly compromise the appetite for and the potential pleasure of sexual activity.

A Gallup survey sponsored by the North American Menopause Society and published in early 1994 polled a random sample of 833 women ages forty-five to sixty, in order to gather information about the women's knowledge of, experience with, and attitudes about menopause and hormone replacement therapy. (I wish that they had polled a random sample of 833 physicians as well, since I have to wonder how many doctors know the facts about testosterone.) The women surveyed provided the following statistics:

Only 20 percent believed that a woman's body produces androgens (assuming the women knew that androgens are the family of hormones that includes testosterone).

Of that 20 percent, one woman in four believed that the production of androgens decreases after menopause. In other words, only five women out of one hundred answered in a way that indicated they knew a woman's body normally produces testosterone and that the production of testosterone decreases after menopause. The women who "knew" about testosterone were not asked whether they knew what the functions of testosterone might be, or what the effects might be when it decreases.

The authors of the article reporting these results—recognized experts in gynecology and menopause—are Dr. Isaac Schiff, professor of gynecology at Harvard Medical School and chief of the Women's Care Division at Massachusetts General Hospital, and Dr. Wulf H. Utian, professor and chairman of the Department of Reproductive Biology at Case Western Reserve University in Cleveland. In their comments on the results of the survey, Drs. Schiff and Utian emphasized the need for educating physicians as well as menopausal women about the use of supplementary testosterone:

> The majority of women have heard about estrogen and progestins, with minority reflecting knowledge

about androgens. This parallels physicians' current prescribing habits and is not unexpected. These data reflect lack of physician knowledge or information about androgen and [demonstrate] another area for improved provider and consumer education.

If a woman consulted her doctor about unexplained rapid weight loss, excessive thirst, and frequent urination, the physician would probably consider the possibility that the patient was suffering from diabetes. If urine and blood tests confirmed a diagnosis of diabetes, and if insulin were indicated, the doctor would prescribe the insulin, carefully adjusting the dosage to the patient's particular needs. Insulin deficiency is a life-threatening condition.

If, on the other hand, a premenopausal or menopausal woman manages to tell her doctor that she has lost her familiar experience of sexual desire and vital energy and is "just not feeling like herself," what are the chances that she will be asked about any loss of sensation in her clitoris and nipples? Will her blood testosterone level be determined and, in the event of testosterone deficiency, will the doctor offer to prescribe testosterone, judiciously adjusting the dosage to her particular needs?

I am afraid we know the answer.

The Gallup survey showed that about two-thirds of the women reported that their doctors had not asked about changes they might be experiencing in their sexual functioning. Since many women are uncomfortable about raising these issues with their doctors, the result is that sexual problems are just never mentioned.

Testosterone deficiency is a quality-of-life-threatening condition.

When I asked one clinical researcher about her speculation as to the general ideological resistance to the use of testosterone by women, she said, resignedly, "People think that if you give a male sex hormone to a woman, you'll turn her into a man."

Testosterone is also a female sex hormone.

In May of 1993, I asked a panel of expert clinicians at a Boston meeting of the North American Menopause Society about their practices of prescribing supplementary testosterone for women who show signs and symptoms of deficiency. All but one member of the panel reported clinical experience with testosterone supplements for women. This doctor, an acknowledged expert in hormone supplemental therapy, was silent. When I pressed him for a response, he hesitantly offered that he did not feel comfortable recommending testosterone for women "for reasons that I am afraid are not rationally based." At least he was honest.

Too often the resistance to prescribing supplementary testosterone for a woman suffering symptoms of deficiency boils down to a rigid holding to the irrational notion that "testosterone for women is *unnatural*."

Sixty-four percent of the women surveyed in the Gallup poll got most of their information about menopause and other women's health issues from sources other than their physicians—from friends, books, and the media. Unfortunately, even some reputedly dependable sources provide little useful information about testosterone for women, or—and worse—offer information that is inaccurate or biased through ignorance and filtered through fear.

Discouraging and typically misleading was the treatment of the subject of the use of supplemental testosterone in the 1993 publication of *Harvard Health Letter's Special Report: Postmenopausal Hormone-Replacement Therapy*. A list of symptoms "sometimes attributed to menopause" includes "loss of sexual desire," but within the body of the twenty-six-page document, only one paragraph addresses the use of testosterone. I was dismayed to find this confusing, inaccurate, and negatively biased statement:

> Also on the market are oral drugs that combine estrogens with androgens, or male sex hormones. The ovaries normally produce androgens, but this production decreases somewhat with menopause. Some physicians, mainly outside the U.S., have prescribed them for years to increase libido, as well as to improve mood and even to alleviate hot flashes. If taken for a long time, androgens produce facial and body hair. High doses can increase muscle mass and cause the clitoris to enlarge.

Reading along, we might first wonder *why* the physicians who prescribe androgens are "mainly outside the U.S." Then there is an implication that medicine as practiced within the United States protects American women from the possibility of grotesque developments. What woman would want to risk taking a "male sex hormone" that could make her hairy, muscle-bound, and genitally bizarre? The fact is, it is simply untrue that "if taken for a long time, androgens produce facial and body hair." **Only if taken in excessive dosages can testosterone stimulate significant growth of facial and body hair.** A prudent and effective dose of testosterone can be taken by virtually any woman, "for a long time," with no risk of unwanted hair growth. Given the need for accurate information about options for treating testosterone deficiency, this paragraph in as respected a forum as the *Harvard Health Letter* is particularly irresponsible.

Thanks in part to the efforts of Congresswoman Pat Schroeder, there has been significant publicity concerning the lack of quality research in the field of women's health. In the spring of 1992, the Society for the Advancement of Women's Health Research established the *Journal of Women's Health,* and in its inaugural issue, Dr. Anne Colston Wentz wrote in her editorial:

June 18, 1989 was the day that defined women's health research as a legitimate area of discussion. The Government Accounting Office reported . . . that the National Institutes of Health had not monitored the clinical research that they supported to make sure that women were included. . . . Women are responsible for spending two of every three health-care dollars, yet the bulk of research dollars has been spent on male diseases.

I wonder what the history of research and the state of knowledge about testosterone deficiency would be if men suffered the early onset and degree of testosterone deficiency that occur in many women. As it is, in 1994, Alza Pharmaceuticals released a testosterone scrotal skin "patch" for men (in dosages of 4 or 6 milligrams per day, appropriate only for men) for the benefit of those men for whom testosterone supplemental therapy might be indicated. And, in 1997, SmithKline Beecham released a second option for men—a nonscrotal skin patch, also contraindicated for women's use.

In January 1995, *The American Journal of Medicine* published proceedings of a symposium titled "Androgens and Women's Health." This conference, sponsored by the National Institute of Child Health and Human Development, presented twenty-two scientific papers focusing on conditions of testosterone *excess* and on research into the effects of testosterone on metabolism and on ovaries, skin, and hair follicles. Amid all the discussion, there was only one paper— thankfully, a fine one—on testosterone deficiency. I was heartened to find, in the presentation by Drs. Robert Sands and John Studd of Chelsea and Westminster Hospital in London, this clear statement: **"Androgen replacement therapy is a neglected area of medical practice and further research is needed to identify all women who will benefit from it."**

We women who find ourselves at midlife in 1999 would certainly benefit if more definitive studies had already been done on the long-term use of estrogen, progesterone, and testosterone. At the 1993 Boston meeting of the North American Menopause Society, Dr. Rogerio Lobo, professor of ob/gyn at the University of Southern California at Los Angeles, reviewed the statistical results of several epidemiologic studies, which reported that women using adequate supplementary estrogen after menopause *decrease their risk of heart attacks and strokes by at least 50 percent over women not using hormone supplements.* And Dr. J. Christopher Gallagher, professor of medicine at Creighton University Medical School in Omaha, presented statistics showing that *women using adequate supplementary estrogen after menopause reduce their risk of (osteoporotic) bone fractures from 50 percent to 90 percent.*

In November 1994, the results of a three-year study at the NIH known as the PEPI study (which stands for Postmenopausal Estrogen and Progestin Intervention) were released. The full report of the PEPI trial, published in the January 18, 1995, issue of the *Journal of the American Medical Association,* confirms the facts that estrogen can substantially lower the risk of heart disease among postmenopausal women and that adequate progestin prevents the increased risk of cancer of the lining of the uterus. A much larger and longer-term study by the Women's Health Initiative at the NIH will not be completed for another ten years. In April 1995 I spoke to Dr. Loretta P. Finnegan, director of this important and long-awaited research effort, and was disturbed to learn that **the NIH Women's Health Initiative includes no controlled clinical studies on supplemental testosterone for women.**

Following Dr. Finnegan as director is Dr. Susan Hurd, to whom I wrote on September 9, 1997—an excerpt of which follows:

I have recently learned that an additional "arm"—
"the memory study"—has been added to the Women's
Health Initiative. The population of menopausal
women suffering loss of vital energy and libido as a
consequence of testosterone deficiency and choosing
to take physiological dosage of supplemental testosterone is large and growing. I am writing to urge that
you add an "arm" to the Women's Health Initiative to
study the long-term safety of supplemental testosterone. If I can be of use in the implementation of this
process, I will do whatever I can.

I received a response from Dr. Jacques Roussouw, which
concluded:

Because of funding constraints and the fact that en-
rollment is virtually complete, it is not possible to add
another design element in the form of a randomized
trial of testosterone at this stage. We can only hope
that others will take up the challenge to do the research that is needed!

This omission is unconscionable. We need responsible research on the effects and safety of long-term use of estrogen,
progesterone, *and testosterone.*

Those of us at risk who do not wish to allow our bones to
become porous, our arteries to become sclerotic, and our genitals to atrophy are choosing to take supplementary estrogen
in the service of a healthier life. And those of us who develop
a premature loss of vital energy and sexual energy and do not
want to settle for it have a right to expect our doctors to inform
themselves about the physiology and function of testosterone
in women so that they can offer us the option of supplemental testosterone and a better quality of life.

∽ 3 ∾

TESTOSTERONE:

A *female* SEX HORMONE!

"I thought that testosterone was the male *sex hormone."*

In one very particular way, it *is*. In its earliest crucial functions—in the developing embryo—testosterone plays the key role in signaling the cells of the genetically male embryo to develop as a male. As astonishing as it may seem, all human embryos begin as females. For the first few weeks of an embryo's life, a small group of cells have the potential to become either ovaries or testes. Of the approximately one million genes that are needed to direct the development of a human being, one single gene, the "SRY" gene, which is carried on the Y chromosome, is responsible for determining the sex of the baby. If the embryo's cells contain the "SRY" gene, the embryo will develop testes (instead of ovaries), which at a critical point and for a very limited time early in its development produce and release a surge of testosterone. This hormone then signals the cells of other parts of the embryo to develop as a male.

As one research scientist in the Goodfellow Group, the researchers who discovered the "SRY" gene, commented, "I sometimes think it is remarkable that we are talking about [the fact that] a few thousand cells [functioning] for perhaps forty-eight hours during development is all that it takes to convert the female body form into the male body form."

By the time a baby is born, the extra boost of testosterone has long passed, and from birth to puberty girls and boys have about the same low levels of estrogen—and of testosterone.

Did you know that puberty for both girls and boys is "kicked off" by the production of testosterone by the adrenal glands? (Each of a pair of very thin, delicate adrenal glands sits like a sort of "hat" at the top of each kidney.) The outer portion of the adrenal gland, the adrenal cortex, produces a group of hormones of related function, known as androgens, the most potent of which is testosterone. The cortex of the adrenal glands is a virtual hormone factory, producing not only androgens, but also cortisone and other hormones, some of which regulate the immune system, while others regulate salt and water balance. In girls, the adrenal glands begin to produce testosterone earlier than in boys. That's how and why girls mature earlier, as a rule, than boys. Just as the beginning of the menstrual cycle is called menarche, this beginning of adrenal production of androgens is called adrenarche. Similarly, just as there is a menopause, there is also an adrenopause (although the adrenal glands never stop producing androgens altogether).

Did you know that a woman's ovaries primarily produce testosterone, from which estrogen is made? Not all the testosterone becomes estrogen, though. Enough testosterone remains unconverted to estrogen to amount to one-fourth of our daily production of this hormone. Another one-fourth is produced by our adrenal glands, and the remaining half by tissues in many different parts of the body, including the liver, the skin, and the brain. These tissues manufacture testosterone from precursor hormones that are made in the ovaries and the adrenals. In other words, the ovaries and the adrenal glands are responsible for producing *all* of a woman's testosterone— directly or indirectly.

Did you know that men's bodies produce estrogen? Men's tissues convert a small amount of their testosterone into this "female sex hormone." In fact, adult males have about the same amount of estrogen as postmenopausal women.

"What does testosterone do in a woman's body?"

Do you remember what it was like to begin to mature? It was testosterone that stimulated the growth of your pubic hair and underarm hair (there are testosterone receptors in the skin of the pubic area and in the skin of the underarm that are genetically programmed to react to testosterone by producing hair). And testosterone stimulated your skin to produce more oil, contributing to the acne of your early teenage years, but also to the healthy glow of your skin and the shine of your hair.

In addition, there are testosterone receptors in the nipples of the developing breasts, as well as in the clitoris and in the vagina, that make them sensitive to sexual stimulation.

There are receptors *in the brain* that respond to testosterone by establishing the neurochemical basis for the experience of falling in love.

One researcher, curious about the fact that only male canaries sing, gave testosterone to female canaries, who then "burst into song." He was able to trace this change to increased stimulation of an area in the front part of the brain of the canary. Research on humans has demonstrated that testosterone receptors are concentrated in those areas of the brain involved in sex and emotions.

Without testosterone, we would have no pubic hair, no sensitivity to sexual pleasure in the nipples or genitals, and no receptivity to the sexual aspect of falling in love—no capacity to "turn on."

"What else does testosterone do?"

An endocrinologist's bible, the medical textbook *Reproductive Endocrinology*, edited by Drs. Samuel Yen and Robert

Jaffe, states: "Testosterone and other androgens have some biological activity on virtually every tissue in the body." Among the most important functions listed are "anabolic actions, such as stimulation of linear body growth, nitrogen retention, and muscular development." This means that testosterone works to keep the cells of the body functioning efficiently, making the best use of nourishment for growth and maintenance, and particularly contributing to the health of bones and muscles.

With adequate effective testosterone, we have the maximal opportunity to experience our body's innate vital energy and sense of well-being. Without enough effective testosterone, the body develops what physiologists describe as a "catabolic state"—a state in which the maintenance and growth of affected tissues suffer a decline, and in which we experience a loss of muscle tone, vital energy, and sense of well-being.

"How much testosterone does a woman produce, and how much does she need?"

From the "kickoff" of testosterone production at puberty, and as long as women have fully functioning ovaries, their bodies produce, on the average, three-tenths of one milligram of testosterone per day. Men's bodies produce more than twenty times as much, or an average of seven milligrams of testosterone per day.

Testosterone is carried in the blood, most of it attached to a protein known as "sex hormone binding globulin," or SHBG. Only a tiny amount of testosterone is unattached to protein, or "free" in the plasma—free to produce its effects on tissues. Ninety-seven to 99 percent of women's testosterone is attached to protein at any given time. Therefore, only 1 to 3 percent is available to act on tissues.

Both testosterone and estrogen are carried on the same

protein. Estrogen actually stimulates the production of *more* SHBG, which then binds up still more of the testosterone— leaving less testosterone to be *free* to work on cells. (This explains why taking supplementary estrogen at menopause can tie up a little more of whatever testosterone we may still have, sometimes tipping the balance and causing symptoms of testosterone deficiency.)

"What are testosterone 'receptors'?"

Like all hormones (including estrogen), testosterone works by attaching to specific cellular proteins, known as receptors. The cells of some tissues produce more testosterone receptors than others (the cells of the genital area, for example, are abundantly supplied with testosterone receptors). Among the changes that occur in our tissues as we grow older are the gradually diminishing levels of testosterone receptors and the reduction of enzymes that are involved in the utilization of testosterone at the cellular level. While factors in our internal and external environments no doubt play some part, patterns of aging are significantly determined by the genes we inherit.

Sensitivity to testosterone is a variable and not yet completely understood phenomenon. The effect of a particular blood level of testosterone varies from woman to woman. In other words, two women with identical blood testosterone levels may experience different degrees of testosterone effect. The genetically determined differences in the numbers (and distribution in their tissues) of testosterone receptors may be one factor. Because of the variability from woman to woman in the number of testosterone receptors and in the complexity of the hormonal climate (that is, the levels of other hormones as they affect one another), each woman's case must be considered individually. It is more likely that a woman and her doctor will need to tailor a hormone supplement program to meet her particular needs than that any programmed dosage schedule will suit her.

As well, there does not appear to be a simple "dose/response curve" in the use of supplementary testosterone. In other words, the effects of testosterone do not vary directly with the dose of testosterone given. By no means is it true that if some is good, more is better when it comes to the effectiveness of supplementary testosterone. Many women benefit more from a lower effective dose of testosterone than from a higher dose.

Research has shown, *definitively,* that raising the level of testosterone above a normal range level does not stimulate further increase in sexual energy. Women who have taken more than a physiologic dose (a dose equivalent to what the body normally produces) of testosterone have told me that they did not feel sexier and better. Rather, if they felt anything in particular, they felt more irritable (even agitated), easily provoked to anger, and hungrier for food. One woman reported that she woke up in the middle of the night, "hyper" and wide awake, but not sexually aroused. She added, "There was no chance that I could go back to sleep. This was not insomnia. It was three A.M. and I was up for the day."

With most hormones, strong reactions to initial high blood levels can smooth out over time. But even if a woman "gets used to" a level of testosterone above the normal physiologic range, there are several reasons why continuing to take a high level is not desirable.

For one thing, testosterone is inactivated by the liver, where metabolism of the testosterone can interfere with production of HDL (high-density lipoproteins, or "good cholesterol"). Moreover, if a woman maintains abnormally high blood levels of testosterone over a period of time (which I believe is medically irresponsible), she may develop acne, increased downy facial hair, and, in extreme cases, a lowering of her voice. These symptoms of excessive testosterone use are known as virilizing side effects.

There is no justification for any woman to take a dose of testosterone high enough to cause virilizing side effects.

I have experienced a "lag time" in my body's response to changing the dose of testosterone upward or downward. The exact scientific basis for this phenomenon, observed by several researchers as well, has not yet been demonstrated, but the fact that it may take several weeks for a woman to experience the full effect of any dose level is important information for her and her doctor to know.

The amount of testosterone, tiny as it is, that a woman's body is continually producing is an *essential* amount. There is a critical point, which appears to vary somewhat from woman to woman for the complex of factors we have just mentioned, at which less available testosterone results in symptoms of *deficiency*. If your testosterone drops below the critical point for you, you will notice a loss of vital energy and feeling of well-being. You will experience a loss of your familiar level of sexual desire, your nipples and genitals will become less sensitive, and your pubic hair might become thinner in texture and sparser. You will experience a "flatness" of mood and might notice some loss of mental sharpness. You might develop dry skin and brittle scalp hair. You will notice some loss of muscle tone. Other effects of testosterone deficiency can include decreased production of red blood cells by bone marrow and loss of calcium from bones, which can contribute to osteoporosis.

Testosterone deficiency may also contribute to the loss of muscle tone in the bladder and pelvis, resulting in symptoms of urinary incontinence. (Other possible causes of urinary incontinence include infection, anatomic defects, and cardiovascular-renal disease, which must be ruled out or treated appropriately if present.) Women who need and use supplementary testosterone, conceivably in conjunction with Kegel exercises (contracting and relaxing inner pelvic muscles), have a maximal opportunity for maintaining bladder sphincter tone.

*"I've always had quite a lot of body hair. Does this mean that
I have more testosterone than my friend, who never needs a
'bikini wax'?"*

Women whose bodies produce a normal level of testosterone
can develop different amounts of body hair, depending upon
the genes they have inherited that influence the degree of activity of a particular skin enzyme, known as 5-alpha-reductase.
Research has shown that most women who are by nature
"hairy" have more of this enzymatic activity in their skin than
women who are less "hairy."

*"I've seen articles about an endocrine condition where the
woman has too much testosterone and excessive body hair."*

In 1935, Drs. Stein and Leventhal observed some women to
have signs and symptoms, such as the lack of menstrual periods, excessive body hair, obesity, and ovaries enlarged by multiple cysts, that indicated a metabolic disorder they named
polycystic ovary syndrome, or PCO. Though the label of PCO
has stuck, it is now recognized that the disorder may have
nothing to do with cystic ovaries! I found the most intelligent,
clear, and full discussion of this poorly understood condition
in Yen and Jaffe's *Reproductive Endocrinology* text, in which
Dr. Yen explains that the onset of PCO syndrome is *at puberty.* Most probably under genetic control, the level of activity of enzymes crucial to the normal production of androgens
by the adrenal glands and by the ovaries becomes elevated.
This results in the excessive production of these androgens,
and shows up as excessive body-hair growth, irregularity of
menstrual periods, and overweight.

Dr. Yen stresses that a woman who has developed normally at puberty and sometime later develops, relatively
rapidly, excessive body hair, acne, and menstrual irregularities
"requires urgent and special diagnostic methods for distin-

guishing the PCO syndrome from other more serious causes of androgen excess." These "other more serious causes" are not common, and can include androgen-secreting tumors and potentially life-threatening malfunctions of the adrenal glands. PCO syndrome itself can present complex hormonal abnormalities, including excessive estrogen production and problems with sugar metabolism.

In addition, the complex of glandular malfunctions in PCO syndrome always results in infertility. Dr. Richard S. Legro of the Department of Ob/Gyn at Pennsylvania State College of Medicine states that "there is no consensus as to the nature of . . . PCO syndrome." This observation is unfortunately true, even though an informed consensus *could* exist. While the metabolic malfunctions are not altogether clear, the basic clinical picture is. Not all hairy women have PCO syndrome. The onset of signs and symptoms at puberty is key. Treatment of PCO syndrome can be approached via a variety of hormone manipulations, including the use of clomiphene. An anti-estrogen (often used in treating infertility from other causes), clomiphene can help a woman suffering from PCO syndrome begin to ovulate, normalize her hormone systems, and establish fertility. Other treatments to control the excess production of androgens can also be used.

It is interesting to note that women diagnosed with PCO syndrome who have blood levels of testosterone above the normal range have not been noted to experience increased libido. This is consistent with my own observations that women dosed excessively with supplementary testosterone do not experience a correspondingly increased libido, but can develop (as do women with PCO syndrome) the "virilizing" side effects of increased body and facial hair and acne.

The treatment of disorders of androgen excess includes the option of using drugs that shut off or block the actions of androgens, though such a treatment can result in a woman's developing symptoms of testosterone deficiency. Dr. Florence Haseltine of the NIH has cautioned, with regard to the use of "androgen blocking agents," that "therapy should be individualized according to the patient's appearance, psychosocial problems, sexual function, childbearing decisions, and enhanced risk of other diseases." She goes on to say, "While no single medical treatment is appropriate for all manifestations of androgen-excess abnormalities, all therapy should be based on a physiologic understanding of the underlying problem and a sensitivity to the woman's needs and concerns."

How wonderful it would be if all therapy for any imbalance or illness *were* based on a physiologic understanding of the underlying problem and a sensitivity to the woman's needs and concerns. Certainly, as regards conditions of testosterone deficiency or excess, this paradigm is especially important.

"I'm two years past menopause and my libido has fallen off, but I don't notice any loss of pubic hair. Could I be testosterone deficient?"

Yes. Some women who develop symptoms of loss of energy and libido when their testosterone drops below a critical level may continue to have the same amount of pubic hair they had previously, due to genetically determined higher levels of skin enzyme (5-alpha-reductase) activity.

"Since menopause, my genital tissue has become very fragile. Estrogen hasn't helped. My doctor says I have something called 'LSA,' and that testosterone might help. What does this mean?"

LSA stands for lichen sclerosis atrophicus—a condition of the skin of the vulva that occurs most commonly in postmenopausal women, but also can occur to the genital skin of men and of young children—whereby the skin loses its elasticity, can develop pale white areas, and can atrophy. Recent studies have shown that LSA is due to reduced activity of the same skin enzyme (5-alpha-reductase) responsible for the growth and maintenance of pubic and other body hair.

The late Dr. Eduard Friedrich, Jr., former chairman of the Department of Ob/Gyn at the University of Florida in Gainesville and one of the founding Fellows of the International Society for the Study of Vulvar Disease, published a leading article in 1984 in *The New England Journal of Medicine* describing his research into the cause and treatment of LSA. Dr. Friedrich showed that women who develop LSA also have significantly decreased levels of testosterone—and that most benefit substantially from using testosterone ointment directly on their genital tissue. A full discussion of this method, its advantages and cautions, will be found in Chapter 8 of this book.

*"I've heard of another adrenal androgen called DHEA.
What's that?"*

DHEA stands for dehydroepiandrosterone, a hormone which, together with its sulfated form (DHEA-sulfate, or DS), is the most abundant steroid secreted by the adrenal glands. DHEA and DS are known to decline substantially with age. A fifty-year-old man has less than one-half the DHEA he had at age twenty; a fifty-year-old woman has less than one-third the DHEA she had at age nineteen. Unlike testosterone, DHEA appears to make little direct contribution to libido. Although the function of DHEA is not yet fully known, it appears to have vital importance in keeping the metabolic balance of youth (anabolism), as contrasted with the "wearing out" metabolism of old age (catabolism).

Dr. Yen, who wrote the chapter in *Reproductive Endocrinology* giving the lowdown on DHEA, notes that papers have been published showing the "protective effects of

DHEA on diabetes, cancer, aging and autoimmune diseases in experimental animals," as well as evidence that men with higher levels of DHEA/DS have less heart and vascular disease, women with higher levels of DHEA/DS are at less risk for breast cancer, and both men and women with higher levels of DHEA/DS show evidence of having better-functioning immune systems as they grow older.

In 1994, Dr. Yen and his research associates reported the results of a clinical trial of DHEA therapy that was undertaken with a group of healthy men and women aged forty to seventy. A dose of DHEA was given to the subjects once each day, orally, sufficient to restore a "youthful" blood level of the hormone. The men and women who took the hormone reported "a remarkable increase in perceived physical and psychological well-being, and no change in libido." The researchers did chemical analyses of esoteric-sounding elements that make up something called the GH-IGF-I system, and were able to confirm the action of DHEA in supporting growth and healthy maintenance of tissues in the men and women participating in the study.

Drs. William Regelson, Mohammed Kalimi, and Roger Loria of the Medical College of Virginia consider DHEA to be the "mother steroid"—one that watches over, supports, and regulates the functions of other steroids in their immune system activity (hormones are steroids). Their view is that DHEA will eventually be as widely known as cortisone is today, and that it may prove superior to cortisone in causing fewer undesirable side effects. The idea that supplementary DHEA could be a tonic for our immune system and an aid in keeping ourselves more youthfully healthy as we grow older is exciting to consider.

Attention to testosterone deficiency is one aspect of a breakthrough in medical knowledge. We are at the verge of having enough understanding of cellular physiology and the function of genes to someday influence even the processes of aging. Clinical experience with DHEA today is about where testosterone was fifty years ago. I have found several naturopathic physicians who are prescribing DHEA for their patients, in spite of the fact that very limited and mixed anecdotal information is available as to dosage, long-term safety, and effects. The possibility that DHEA may be an elixir of youth for both men and women is apparently sufficiently compelling to override caution for these practitioners and patients.

It is probable that in the foreseeable future we will have, as part of our routine medical checkups, tests to measure the function of hormones, hormone carriers, enzymes, and receptor sites, as well as the means to adjust these functions. At the present time, though, we do know that testosterone receptor function degenerates more quickly when there is a deficiency of testosterone, and so for this reason, a woman who has symptoms of testosterone deficiency and plans to use supplementary testosterone might "protect her receptors" by using supplemental testosterone sooner than later.

4

TESTOSTERONE DEFICIENCY AND MENOPAUSE

By the time we begin to have signs that our ovaries are shutting down, we have had a significant part of our adult lives to get to know ourselves and the way we function sexually and energetically. If we're lucky, we will have made peace with our sexual rhythms, our patterns of intimacy with our partners, and our psychosexual complexity—or, in other words, what works for us sexually.

For the past twenty-five years, my work as a psychiatrist has taught me to appreciate the differences, substantial and subtle, in the ways we experience and practice the intimate and sexual aspects of life. Sexual desire is influenced by many factors—relational, situational, psychological, and physical. The following comments, written in response to an anonymous questionnaire that was answered by several hundred women at workshops I have taught, are representative of observations women make about the loss of libido.

From a forty-nine-year-old woman who is still having menstrual periods: "I've been wondering if my libido is diminished over the last year or so—but this question has been occurring to me at the same time I'm grieving the loss of my mother, so I'm not sure what is happening right now."

A fifty-five-year-old woman, whose last period occurred at age fifty-two, writes: "I am wondering if my body is telling me that my partner of five years is not 'the one.' "

A forty-six-year-old woman who is still menstruating comments: "I don't think about having sex. I wonder whether this is hormonally related or psychological, because my husband and I have problems with having sex."

A forty-seven-year-old woman, also premenopausal, notes: "I had/have chronic fatigue syndrome—an extenuating circumstance that makes it hard to evaluate the loss of libido I am experiencing."

And a fifty-year-old whose last period was a year ago writes: "I've been exhausted, overworked. I'd rather sleep— or at least that's my excuse. But really I'm just not interested."

Whatever other factors may be playing a part in a woman's loss of interest in making love, without adequate testosterone, sexual desire simply cannot exist. In other words, we are more at the mercy of our hormones for our experience of sexual desire than we might wish to believe. Particularly for women whose loss of interest in sex makes them (or their partners) wonder "whether this means that the love is gone," knowing that the problem might be testosterone deficiency could prevent a considerable amount of potentially unnecessary anguish.

"Why do some women develop testosterone deficiency around the time of menopause?"

During our mid- to late teens our adrenal glands produce peak amounts of testosterone and other androgens. Even before most of us begin to approach menopause, during our mid- to late thirties our adrenal androgen production decreases by more than half. This is the "adrenopause" I referred to earlier, and reflects the decline in DHEA and DS I previously discussed. Our adrenal glands continue to produce some androgens throughout our lifetime, but the amount produced is greatly reduced—down to 18 percent of original production after age seventy. When our ovaries shut down, the amount of testosterone they produce is reduced by one-half. Since both our adrenal glands and ovaries are the source for the building blocks of testosterone that are produced by other tissues, when the ovaries and adrenals slow their production, the end result is a significant reduction in overall testosterone.

Research has shown that in order for a woman's adrenal glands to produce their maximal amount of androgens, her ovaries have to be well functioning. The fact that the workings of the adrenal cortex is linked to the workings of the ovary may be a consequence of a fascinating fact: In the developing embryo, one original group of cells is the source both for the ovaries (or testes) *and* for the outer parts of the adrenal glands. As the embryo develops, these cells actually migrate to the two locations, some of them forming the ovaries (or testes) and others forming the outer parts of the adrenal glands.

If a woman of any age—even a nineteen-year-old, whose adrenals are at peak androgen production—should have her ovaries removed surgically (or functionally destroyed by chemotherapy), *her adrenal glands will subsequently produce less androgens.* She will lose not only all of her ovarian estrogen, progesterone, and testosterone, but also a portion of her adrenal testosterone and other androgens.

The bottom line is that we need fully functioning ovaries in order to maintain fully functioning adrenals.

While men's adrenal glands also show a drop in androgen production with aging, the drop is less precipitous. The difference is probably due to the continued function of the testes, which, unlike the ovaries, do not shut down dramatically at midlife.

Before I did the research, I knew that the average age for a woman at menopause is about fifty. I was surprised to learn that 8 percent of all women have a full, natural menopause before the age of forty. Symptoms of testosterone deficiency can develop for these women as early as their mid- to late thirties.

"I went through menopause at age fifty-one. My mid- to late thirties was the time that felt like my sexual prime. How do you explain that?"

The short answer is that at that time, with this person's particular balance of hormonal factors, she had more available testosterone.

During the years just before menopause, often called the peri-menopause, the ovaries produce estrogen but often fail to mature an egg follicle. This means that the ovaries fail to ovulate, and so fail to produce progesterone, which is made by the follicle cells of the ripening egg.

Another element in this complex tapestry of hormonal interactions is that for 50 percent of women, when the ovaries stop producing eggs, the ovarian tissue (ovarian *stroma*) that produces testosterone responds to the pituitary gland's attempt to get it to ovulate by producing *more* testosterone. When this happens, a woman may experience some increase or return of vital energy and libido. How long this level of testosterone effect may last depends on the rate at which testosterone production by the adrenals and ovaries continues to decrease, as well as on the genetically determined receptor and enzyme factors discussed previously.

Researchers have discovered that for about 50 percent of women, the ovaries do not make a major contribution to testosterone production following menopause. These may be the same women who suffer a significant loss of libido following menopause.

Dr. Barbara Sherwin of McGill University in Montreal is a leading researcher in testosterone supplemental therapy for menopausal women, and with regard to the potential increase in the ovaries' production of testosterone at menopause, explains: "When it occurs, this increase in ovarian testosterone production is time limited, so that eventually, testosterone levels decrease in all women."

What is evident is that Margaret Mead, who touted "post-menopausal zest," was conceivably reflecting her own experience and the experience of *some* but by no means *all* postmenopausal women.

"When can a woman develop testosterone deficiency?"

During the two or three years preceding menopause and through the five years following, a significant number (roughly 50 percent) of women who approach menopause naturally—that is, with their uterus and ovaries intact—notice some symptoms of testosterone deficiency. For some women the onset of symptoms of diminished sexual interest and response may be rather sudden—over a period of a few months. For others, the change may be more gradual—over a period of several years.

A gradual development of testosterone deficiency is a function of aging for all women, as a consequence of several factors: loss of ovarian testosterone, diminished production of adrenal androgens, aging testosterone receptors, and reduced enzyme function. Just as there is a wide spectrum of ages at which women experience menopause, there is a wide spectrum of ages at which women develop critical reductions in adrenal androgens and in testosterone receptor and enzymatic failure. Some women have the genetic predisposition to maintain androgen production and receptor and enzyme functions adequate to keep them vital for decades longer than others.

Nearly one-half of the women who have their ovaries removed (most often accompanying hysterectomy), no matter what their age, are likely to develop testosterone deficiency precipitously, due to the total loss of ovarian testosterone together with the reduction in adrenal androgens that follows the total loss of ovarian function. In spite of increasing awareness that most hysterectomies are avoidable, hysterectomy continues to be the second most frequently performed major surgical procedure in the United States (surpassed only by cesarean section—another often-avoidable procedure). To me, the statistics are horrifying. A recent Gallup survey confirmed that **one-third of American women have their uterus (and too often, their ovaries) removed—most often before the age of fifty.**

In 1995 (the most recent year for which statistics are available from the National Center for Health Statistics) the number of hysterectomies performed in the United States was 583,000—**up** from the 556,000 hysterectomies that had been performed in 1994!

Dr. Vicki Hufnagel, gynecological surgeon and author of the 1988 book with the optimistic title *No More Hysterectomies,* describes in detail the miserable consequences of having one's ovaries removed. She writes about the outrage that "physicians blithely told their patients that the uterus and ovaries had nothing to do with sex" and goes on to affirm that, following hysterectomy, "indeed, the loss of sexuality can be very real." Acknowledging the ovaries as a major source of testosterone, she recognizes that "androgens, in the form of testosterone, enhance women's libido . . . by increasing susceptibility to psychosexual stimulation, heightening sensitivity of the external genitals, and creating greater intensity in sexual gratification."

My experience with women who have had a hysterectomy and have consulted me after developing testosterone deficiency has been heartbreaking. I received an impassioned letter from a forty-nine-year-old woman who had her uterus and ovaries removed because of ovarian cysts and endometriosis when she was thirty-five. She wrote of "utter rage at discovering that [she had] been denied the benefits, or even the *mention,* of testosterone information . . . by more than thirty gynecologists, endocrinologists, internists, psychiatrists, psychopharmacologists, dermatologists, and a few holistic gurus."

During the fourteen years since the removal of her ovaries, she has suffered "dramatic emotional/physical changes." She described a profound loss of sexual desire, thinning and loss of pubic hair, skin rashes and dryness, "little muscle tone and inability to control [her] weight."

Before the surgery, she was an energetic and focused person, "was never late," and "read at least two books a week." She wrote that, following the removal of her ovaries (and while receiving continuous estrogen replacement therapy), "the only way I can describe how I feel about almost everything is that: I either don't care, or I'm too tired to care. It's no longer clear to me which is which. This is a drastic change from how I used to function, and it's difficult to distinguish whether it is from diminished sense of well-being, or having no energy." She goes on to describe herself as "constantly late, disorganized, tak[ing] forever to get ready, tak[ing] three hours to read a newspaper."

This unhappy woman has consulted many doctors over the years, and at various times has been treated with a total of seven different antidepressants and even with lithium (a drug most commonly used to treat manic-depressive illness). "I have constantly been on some drug to get me going since the hysterectomy, but most were a nightmare."

Unfortunately, her story is far from unique. Even today, most women who undergo a hysterectomy with removal of their ovaries are offered *estrogen alone,* if indeed they are offered any hormonal supplements at all after surgery. Too few women are given the option of using supplementary testosterone, even though research conducted over a period of several decades by Drs. Barbara Sherwin and Morrie Gelfand of Montreal has shown that women who are treated with both estrogen and testosterone following a hysterectomy achieve an optimal balance of sexual energy and vital energy, as compared with women given either no hormones or estrogen alone.

Research has shown that **women who have had a hysterectomy leaving their ovaries intact can expect to go through menopause four years earlier, on the average, than they would have had they not had their uterus removed.** The exact cause of this earlier menopause is not known for certain, though Dr. Hufnagel explains that removal of the uterus can lead to ovarian failure as a result of interference with the blood supply to the ovaries. (The uterine artery may be the source for up to two-thirds of the ovaries' blood supply, and surgical removal of the uterus disrupts this source.)

The uterus also produces chemicals, known as prostaglandins, that provide hormonal cyclic stimulation to the ovaries. If the uterus is removed, this rhythm is disrupted, which may be another factor contributing to an earlier menopause. This, in turn, can result in the earlier development of testosterone deficiency.

Women who have been treated with chemotherapy and subsequently experience a "chemical menopause" suffer the same onset of symptoms as women who have had their ovaries removed. In her article in the spring 1992 issue of the *Journal of Sex and Marital Therapy* entitled "A Neglected Issue: The Sexual Side Effects of Current Treatments for Breast Cancer," the late Dr. Helen Singer Kaplan, noted New York sexologist, pointed out that women whose ovaries are functionally wiped out by chemotherapy develop testosterone deficiency, usually without any acknowledgment of the problem, much less any warning beforehand that it could happen.

If a woman has had chemotherapy as a treatment for a non-hormone-sensitive cancer, such as lymphoma, the use of supplemental testosterone for symptoms of deficiency could safely restore vital energy and libido. If the cancer was potentially hormone-sensitive (breast, ovarian, uterine), the decision about supplemental use of estrogen and/or testosterone is a tougher call to make. Definitive risk/benefit data is not available, and cancer specialists are not of one mind as to what to recommend.

It concerns me that several of the best papers published on the subject of testosterone deficiency focus on women who have no ovarian function, either as a result of the surgical removal of their ovaries or as a result of the loss of ovarian function due to chemotherapy for cancer. This narrow pathologizing of testosterone deficiency has a distorting effect. To be sure, women who have developed testosterone deficiency as a result of surgery or of chemotherapy need attention to their problems, but *many women who develop testosterone deficiency are women with intact ovaries, who have never had chemotherapy, and who develop this deficiency—sometimes even before menopause—as a result of their constitutional predisposition.*

In the same way that estrogen deficiency is an aspect of normal menopause, we could say that testosterone deficiency is an aspect of normal menopause and aging. The fact that it is a "normal" part of the aging process, however, does not mean that it should be ignored any more than should the gradual onset of osteoporosis or any other treatable condition.

Just as estrogen deficiency can be treated with supplemental estrogen, testosterone deficiency can be treated with supplemental testosterone. Physicians are learning to recognize the signs and symptoms of estrogen deficiency, as well as the considerations for treating it. That is all to the good.

Physicians must learn to ask about symptoms, look for signs, learn about potential treatment of testosterone deficiency in peri-menopausal and aging women, and get that information out to those who need it.

5

RECOGNIZING

TESTOSTERONE DEFICIENCY

"How do I know if I have enough testosterone?"

The most obvious signs of testosterone deficiency are:

1. Overall decreased sexual desire.
2. Diminished vital energy and sense of well-being.
3. Decreased sensitivity to sexual stimulation in the clitoris.
4. Decreased sensitivity to sexual stimulation in the nipples.
5. Overall decreased arousability and capacity for orgasm.
6. Thinning and loss of pubic hair (in some women).

Certainly, each woman must evaluate her sexual arousability in the full context of her physical, emotional, historical, and relational circumstances.

Here are the questions to ask yourself in evaluating the possibility that your body may not be producing sufficient testosterone:

1. What is my familiar level of vital energy, sense of well-being, sexual desire, and pleasure?

2. Am I suffering a significant loss in this familiar level of energy, well-being, sexual desire, and pleasure?
3. Do I particularly notice a lack of arousability in my nipples and clitoris?
4. Do I notice not only that I have no particular interest in making love, but also (if this has been a part of your sexual life) that I do not feel like masturbating?
5. In even the most conducive-to-me circumstances, does it take a long time for me to be aroused?
6. If I do have an orgasm, is it diminished in intensity?
7. Have I noticed (if this has a been part of your sexual life) a lack of sexual dreams or sexual fantasies?

Each of us has her own particular adjustment to the sexual aspect of life, with her own familiar rhythms of sexual feelings, fantasies, dreams, and activities. The answers to these questions must be considered in the full context of your personal sexual history and your present circumstances.

We all know that life circumstances can certainly disrupt sexual rhythms, but the "wipeout" of sexual desire that results from a critical reduction in testosterone is different from the fluctuations we experience with the various ups and downs of life and relationships. If your level of testosterone drops below a critical point, which may occur several years before menopause, your familiar levels and expressions of sexual desire may drop off notably, sometimes over a period of only a few months. This occurrence is most apparent for women whose other life circumstances remain stable.

A common concern among women who have been previously satisfied with their intimate relationships, in the face of the radical loss of sexual desire, is expressed in the question "Can this mean that I really don't love my partner?" And the partners of women who suffer a hormonal loss of sexual desire express their anguish as well. As one husband said, "I felt she was no longer in love with me. We made love occasionally, but it was not the same at all. As I got the cold shoulder, I got less and less likely to even try."

Referring to her experience prior to using supplementary testosterone, one woman who consulted me said, "I had absolutely no libido. In fact, I had not had a climax for a year, and I was becoming very depressed. I started to wonder if something was seriously wrong, like did I have cancer."

On a workshop questionnaire, a woman wrote: "I used to be easily aroused, and had frequent ejaculatory orgasms. Now I am not easily aroused by either thoughts (as before) or my lover. Orgasms are rarely wet, and intercourse is painful."

Another woman wrote: "I always considered myself to have a very strong libido. Now it seems that sex does not matter."

Another: "I just don't feel like myself. I never knew I could feel so 'dead' sexually."

And another: "I feel like an incomplete woman, because I have no libido anymore."

These expressions are echoed, with variations on a theme, by too many women—women going through or past natural menopause, women who have had their ovaries removed surgically, women who have lost ovarian function due to chemotherapy, and even women who have had an illness, or have taken medication, that has affected brain chemistry or hormonal balance.

Several women who contacted me after reading my letter to the *New York Times* reported symptoms of testosterone deficiency triggered by unusual circumstances. One woman was poisoned by exposure to phenol in her workplace when she was forty years old. Before this devastating misfortune, she had been healthy, was still menstruating regularly, and was enjoying "a great sex life." Three years later, she was struggling with slowly resolving residual neurological effects, including problems with her vision and visual memory. These symptoms troubled her, but she complained even more bitterly about her lack of general vital energy and sexual libido. She was still menstruating, but had noticed a substantial loss of pubic hair. She contacted me, complaining, "I just don't feel like myself."

It was not surprising, given all of her symptoms, that her blood testosterone levels proved to be very low. She opted to use supplementary testosterone, and has kept in touch to let me know that it has restored her to a level of energy, desire, and pleasure that has helped her feel more like herself again.

While it is possible that the hormonal changes that this woman experienced might have occurred even without the disaster of the phenol poisoning, it is also possible that the testosterone deficiency may have developed as a consequence of disruption of the balance and production of pituitary, adrenal, and ovarian hormones and of brain chemical messengers (neurotransmitters) that resulted from the poisoning. Whatever the cause, she has shown much improvement as a result of using supplementary testosterone.

An extraordinary request for consultation came from a Connecticut woman in her early fifties who identified herself as being transsexual. She was born a physically normal male and, at age twenty-eight underwent a sex-change operation with surgical removal of both testes. In order to develop and maintain female bodily attributes (breasts, fat distribution patterns, and higher voice register), she has been taking large doses of estrogen since she was twenty-three. It is inevitable that, without testicles and with the drop in the adrenal hormones that accompanies that loss, she has been experiencing symptoms of testosterone deficiency—lack of energy, sexual desire, and pleasure—for many years.

The options available in this circumstance are tricky. One issue is her concern about the risk that supplementary testosterone might stimulate the growth of facial hair. If she were to take enough testosterone to bring her blood level into the normal male range, this could happen. The hair-forming elements (PSU's, or "pilosebaceous units") in her facial skin are genetically programmed to respond to normal male levels of testosterone by growing stubbly beard hair. Once a beard has been established genetically and hormonally, only electrolysis, which destroys the hair follicles, can permanently do away with it. Women who take physiological doses of testosterone do not have to be concerned about "growing a beard," because our facial PSU's are not genetically programmed to do that. Instead, we grow fine, downy facial hair, which, so long as we maintain a blood level of testosterone in the normal female range, cannot become stubbly beard hair.

With regard to this transsexual woman's dilemma, the question remains as to whether taking a supplemental dose of testosterone that would be enough to raise her blood level to the top of the female range would stimulate any significant improvement in her vital energy or sexual libido and sensation. Since a man has more testosterone receptors in his brain and the rest of his body and needs seven to ten times more testosterone than a woman in order to maintain his energy and sexual libido, a major improvement for this woman who was originally created male is doubtful. Given the fact that her testosterone receptors are profoundly depleted, she might obtain some benefit from a low dose of testosterone, low enough not to restimulate a deep voice, male hair-growth patterns, and muscle mass. She is thinking things over, as yet undecided about what may be worth trying.

"Can men develop testosterone deficiency?"

Because most men's testes continue to produce significant levels of testosterone as they age, and their adrenal androgens maintain at substantial levels longer than women's, the majority of healthy men experience only a gradual and moderate decline in vital energy and sexual libido as they grow older. Of course, some men, with the genetic disposition, general health, and life circumstances favoring it, continue to be vigorous energetically and sexually well into older age. Other men's genes, health, and life circumstances lead to earlier failure in testosterone production by the testes and the adrenals, resulting in the loss of libido and vital energy at an earlier age. On the basis of inadequate levels of testosterone, some men become functionally impotent.

Epidemiological studies show that, while most men in their fifties and sixties will notice some reduction in energy and sexual vigor, it is unusual for a man in his forties or fifties to experience the total bottoming-out of testosterone with the loss of vital energy and sexual libido that occurs in many women.

Dr. Edward Klaiber is an endocrinologist in private practice and a research scientist formerly at the Worcester Foundation for Experimental Biology in Shrewsbury, Massachusetts—the labs where Dr. Gregory Pincus developed the Pill. (Coincidentally, in 1959, during the summer between my sophomore and junior years at Wellesley College, I had my first exposure to endocrinological research when I worked at the Worcester Foundation as a research assistant to the late Dr. Harris Rosenkrantz, studying the effects of vitamin E deficiency on the adrenal glands of rabbits.)

Dr. Klaiber's clinical research for the past twenty-five years has been focused on studying the effects of supplementary estrogen and testosterone for both women and men. In talking with Dr. Klaiber, I learned that there has actually been more clinical research conducted over the past forty years in treating women with supplementary testosterone than there has been in treating men!

I have also reviewed a very interesting series of papers published by a group under the direction of John B. McKinlay at the New England Research Institute. A study funded by the National Institutes of Health and Aging, called the Massachusetts Male Aging Study, has completed a survey of seventeen hundred men aged forty to seventy who were recruited at random from the greater Boston community. At the launch of the survey, an early publication by these researchers observed that "methodological problems [rendered] earlier work on women of limited value." Based on my own review of the medical literature, I can confirm that many studies of aging women have been very poorly designed and often reported on too few subjects not chosen at random. The Massachusetts Male Aging Study was determined not to repeat these confounding errors—and certainly did examine "a carefully selected representative sample of normally aging men."

While the research group did succeed in carefully collecting some quite interesting data, it's the way in which they *interpreted* this data that I find of greater interest. In an initial paper (in 1989), McKinlay and his co-authors emphasize the idea that "considerable controversy exists about steroid hormone levels and aging men, and *if such a condition as the 'male climacterium' [male 'menopause'] exists [my emphasis].*" The premise of this early paper is a challenge to the possibility that aging men have reduced hormone levels and may have reduced sexual functioning on that basis.

As the results of the study came in, there could be no doubt that aging men were found both to have reduced testosterone levels and reduced sexual functioning. The final paper reported by that research group in 1994 focused particularly on the incidence of impotence in their aging population, showing that the incidence of complete impotence tripled from 5 percent at age forty to 15 percent at age seventy, and that "moderate impotence" doubled from 17 percent at age forty to 34 percent at age seventy. The authors concluded that "impotence is a major health concern in light of the high prevalence" and that it "is strongly associated with age."

In spite of the fact that men's sex hormones decrease as they age and that loss of potency is associated with aging, the authors are reluctant to acknowledge that the loss of potency (in otherwise healthy men) is a function of hormonal decline. At the same time, though, they do recognize that conditions such as vascular disease, hypertension, diabetes, associated medication, cigarette smoking, and alcohol or drug use can cause impotence.

When all is said and done, I am left with the impression that these researchers (and many of the rest of us) simply do not want to believe that men's or women's capacity for sexual pleasure and function is dependent on adequate hormone levels, which decrease over time. As is, of course, true for both men and women, other factors—factors of health, medication, substance use, personality, and personal circumstances—can very substantially influence a person's appetite and capacity for sexual pleasure. But no matter what the other variables, for men as well as for women, without adequate testosterone, sexual desire, sexual pleasure, and sexual function are compromised.

Dr. Klaiber's experience in treating men who come to him complaining of having lost the capacity for sexual desire and pleasure is that about 80 percent of men up to the age of seventy receive significant benefit for this problem from supplementary testosterone. Men with problems of impotence may recover their capacity for erection. Even those for whom full capacity does not return often report a welcome improvement in their desire for sexual contact and in sexual sensitivity and pleasure. Testosterone affects sexual sensitivity in genital tissue for men just as it does for women.

And yet a few cautions exist with regard to supplemental testosterone for men. While there is no evidence that testosterone can cause cancer of the prostate, it is known that it can stimulate the growth of preexisting cancer of the prostate. Dr. Klaiber cautioned that supplementary testosterone can "ignite" an existing cancer that might be dormant or very slow-growing.

For men considering testosterone supplementation, there

is a blood test that can measure prostatic specific antigen, or PSA. It is important to understand that PSA is *not* an indicator of the existence or absence of cancer; it is an indicator of the volume of prostatic tissue. According to Dr. Klaiber, the risk that a very much enlarged prostate (which would produce a larger amount of PSA, in the range of eleven to twenty-two micrograms per liter) might contain an existing cancer is fairly high. Whatever the PSA value, given the fact that the incidence of unsymptomatic cancer of the prostate is very high in older men, the risk of stimulating growth of prostatic cancer in that population must not be disregarded. Still, Dr. Klaiber does not rule out supplementary testosterone for an older man who wants to use it, provided it is carefully prescribed and the man continues to have his PSA monitored. As long as the PSA value remains more or less stable and within safe limits, continued hormone supplementation is a reasonable clinical decision.

"What are the particular benefits and risks of supplementary testosterone for older men and women?"

Dr. Klaiber and I also discussed the potential use of testosterone as an "anabolic tonic" for aging women and men whose testosterone levels may be very low. Elderly people who complain of feeling "worn out," who have little muscle mass, who are frail and cannot gain weight in spite of a good diet, are often depressed about their lack of zest for life and profound lack of energy. A check of their testosterone levels will most often confirm profoundly low levels of total and free testosterone.

Older people who have had major surgery (for illnesses other than cancer) and have difficulty regaining their prior strength and energy may particularly benefit from supplementary testosterone, as may those with chronic heart or lung conditions. Because of the risk of prostatic cancer, though, the potential use of testosterone as a tonic may be safer for aging women than for aging men. Even so, clinical studies of the use and benefit of supplementary testosterone for men in their sixties are under way. I haven't yet heard of any such studies on the benefits of testosterone for aging women.

One of the "tonic" effects of supplementary testosterone is the stimulation of red blood-cell production in the bone marrow. Since elderly men and women have aging and narrowing blood vessels, if the blood becomes "too thick," it could put them at risk for potential heart attack or stroke. Especially considering the dosage of testosterone needed by men, this potentiality needs to be watched by checking the red blood count adequately.

Testosterone also has some natural anticoagulant effect, and is rumored to be "safer than aspirin" in preventing blood clots, heart attack, or stroke. People taking an anticoagulant (such as Coumadin) need to be aware that adding testosterone can further thin their blood.

Since the 1940s, reports have appeared from time to time in the medical literature noting one or another beneficial effect of maintaining adequate testosterone levels. The common thread through these various reports is the observation that adequate levels of testosterone contribute to the health of blood vessels, assuring a better blood supply to the heart muscle, brain, and even to the retina in diabetic patients. What this suggests is that adequate levels of testosterone can help to prevent heart disease, stroke, and diabetic blindness.

To recount a few of these reports:

Researchers at Columbia Medical School reported in 1994 that they had found an inverse correlation between testosterone levels and degree of coronary artery disease. They found that men with higher levels of testosterone have a better blood supply to the heart muscle and higher levels of HDL (the "good" cholesterol) than do men with lower levels of testosterone. Men with lower levels of testosterone have higher degrees of blockage of the coronary arteries and lower levels of HDL.

In an early study, published in 1946, Dr. Maurice Lesser of Boston University School of Medicine reported the results of treating a group of patients suffering from angina pectoris (pain due to inadequate blood supply to the muscle of the heart) with injections of testosterone. He discovered that 91 percent of the group experienced gradual and marked improvement in their cardiac pain.

In 1962, a report appeared in the respected British medical journal *The Lancet* on the benefits of testosterone treatment of patients with occlusive vascular disease—that is, narrowed blood vessels. Serious consequences of this condition can include heart attack, stroke, and, in diabetic patients, severe damage to the retina, possibly leading to blindness. The researchers found that the use of testosterone resulted in significant improvement in this group of patients. They postulated that the beneficial results were the consequence of the blood-thinning properties of testosterone.

In 1964, the *New York State Journal of Medicine* published an article focusing on the complex and vital role of anabolic steroids in regulating blood sugar and insulin requirements in maintaining a healthy metabolic balance. The authors suggested that the benefits of testosterone and of synthetic anabolic steroids in diabetic patients may be due to metabolic improvements at the cellular level, as well as to the blood-thinning effects.

In 1977, the *British Heart Journal* published a report of the work of Dr. Martin Jaffe, who demonstrated that men whose electrocardiogram showed evidence of poorer blood supply to the heart muscle after exercise showed significant improvement after being treated with testosterone.

What is most evident to me from all I have learned in my research is that testosterone is a hormone whose role in the maintenance of health has yet to be fully understood and appreciated. In using supplementary testosterone to maintain our vital energy, sexual energy, and quality of life, we may well be making a significant contribution to our health as well.

For more about the potential cardiovascular protective effects of physiological levels of testosterone, see chapter 8, page 118.

"Is there a way to measure your level of testosterone?"

Yes. There are two methods of measuring your level of testosterone: One tests blood, the other saliva. The best-known and most commonly used method is a blood test, which can measure both total testosterone and unbound, or "free," testosterone (that portion of testosterone that can attach to receptors in the cells and exert its actions). Different methods may be used by different laboratories for these measurements, some more accurate and dependable than others.

My own experience with testosterone determinations has been with tests performed on blood samples. The laboratory I use, Quest Diagnostics (in Cambridge, Massachusetts), reports the normal range of total testosterone to be fourteen to seventy-six nanograms per deciliter. For some perspective on these incredibly tiny amounts: One gram is one-thirtieth of an ounce, one nanogram is one-billionth of a gram, and one deciliter equals about half a cup.

In my view, the "normal" range of blood testosterone levels for women has not been adequately defined. Women with blood levels of total testosterone above fourteen nanograms per deciliter frequently have symptoms of testosterone deficiency. At the other end of the spectrum, it is not common for a woman to have a baseline level of total testosterone of more than fifty nanograms per deciliter. The normal range of total testosterone works out to be something more like twenty to fifty nanograms per deciliter.

Free testosterone is that small percentage (1 to 3 percent) of the total testosterone that is not bound to the carrier protein. The normal range for free testosterone is listed by Quest labs as "one-half to five picograms per milliliter." (One picogram is one-*trillionth* of a gram and one milliliter is one-thirtieth of an ounce, or approximately twenty drops.) Corresponding salivary measurements of free testosterone work out to be about one-tenth the amount found in a matching blood sample—same person, same time.

When a woman reports symptoms of testosterone deficiency, a blood test to measure her total testosterone can sometimes show that she has *no measurable testosterone*. In spite of this, the laboratory data regularly will yield a determination, always very low, for free testosterone. I puzzled over these values before consulting with Dr. Gerald Sheys, technical director of Quest Diagnostics laboratory. I could not understand how the laboratory could come up with a value for free testosterone in a sample reported to have "no measurable total testosterone" in the first place. Dr. Sheys explained that radioimmunoassays for total testosterone cannot measure amounts less than twenty nanograms per deciliter, so that a woman may indeed have an unmeasurable but existent, very small amount of total testosterone. He noted that the blood test used for the free testosterone is a more sensitive test, designed to measure trace amounts, and therefore can detect and measure that tiny percentage of the unmeasurable total testosterone not bound to protein.

Another laboratory mystery presented itself when I was contacted by a woman who was taking Estratest H.S., the most commonly prescribed pharmaceutical combination of methyltestosterone and estrogen. Even though natural testosterone has been available for many years, no preparation of plain testosterone—a natural substance which cannot be patented—is marketed by any drug company. Doctors have remarkable resistance to prescribing anything that is not listed in the *Physicians' Desk Reference* (often referred to as the *PDR*). A major drawback of Estratest H.S. is that, since it exists in the form of a "caplet" containing two hormones in fixed dosage, it does not allow for flexible dosing of one without affecting the dose of the other. I discovered another drawback when this patient's reported testosterone levels proved uninterpretable.

After this woman began taking the Estratest H.S., she experienced improvement in energy, sexual libido, sensation, and orgasm. However, she also developed unpleasant symptoms of agitation and irritability. I suspected that her blood levels of testosterone might be higher than necessary or advisable and suggested a blood test to check this out, but the laboratory results reported "no measurable total testosterone"! The same sample tested for free testosterone reported a value of 4.6 picograms per milliliter—the higher end of the normal range. This simply made no sense. Since the woman was taking a significant dose of supplementary methyltestosterone, her blood should certainly have registered some measurable total testosterone. I had no idea how to interpret the free testosterone value. These results were very puzzling. We repeated the tests, which yielded similar results, and I called Dr. Sheys, the lab director. Upon reviewing the laboratory methodology, and in joint consultation with Dr. Richard Reitz, medical director of the Corning Nichols Laboratory in San Juan Capistrano, California, we discovered that *methyl*testosterone cannot be measured by the standard assay that measures total unmethylated testosterone. A blood test to measure total and free testosterone can yield accurate data *only when the person is not taking methyltestosterone.*

Upon contacting Solvay Pharmaceuticals, the manufacturer of Estratest, I spoke several times to investigators in the Women's Health Clinical Endocrinology Operations section, who acknowledged that Solvay does have a method of measuring methyltestosterone blood levels, but that this method is both highly specialized and "proprietary."

I have learned some important facts about the way the body uses methyltestosterone, leading me to conclude that even if we had a readily available laboratory method of measuring methyltestosterone blood levels, the meaning of these test results would be of somewhat limited use.

1. When methyltestosterone is absorbed from the gut, it is carried by the blood directly to the liver, where 44 percent of it is immediately processed to be excreted.
2. Some of the remaining 56 percent of the methyltestosterone is acted upon by the liver to remove the "methyl" elements, and as the hormone circulates, most of the testosterone (with and without the "methyl") gets bound up to carrier protein.
3. Some small percentage of the testosterone (with and without the "methyl") is free to attach to receptors. The free testosterone that still has the "methyl" **has less affinity for testosterone receptors.** This means that any free methyltestosterone is less clinically active than the free testosterone that has been unmethylated.
4. Unless there was some way to measure both the methylated and unmethylated free testosterone and to know exactly how active the free methyltestosterone can be, we can only estimate the level of testosterone activity at any dosage of methyltestosterone.

What we know for sure is **there is no way to obtain an accurate measurement of the level of testosterone activity a person may have when he or she is taking methyltestosterone.**

"Is the saliva test a better way to measure testosterone?"

A laboratory method that utilizes saliva and measures only free testosterone was developed about seventeen years ago and has been the method of choice of Dr. James M. Dabbs, Jr., a professor and researcher in the Department of Psychology at Georgia State University in Atlanta. Dr. Dabbs believes that salivary measurements in a sample containing methyltestosterone are confounded by the same complex problems that confound attempts at blood measurements, but where methyltestosterone is not an element in the picture, salivary sampling offers several advantages over blood tests for measurement of testosterone levels. In Dr. Dabbs's words:

> To understand fully the relationships between hormones and behavior, we need to know what happens in natural settings outside the laboratory. . . . We have gathered data in settings ranging from bedrooms to barrooms, among subjects who include children, adults, unemployed day laborers, lawyers, prisoners, politicians and two chimpanzees.

The method of saliva collection involves chewing sugar-free gum (to stimulate the flow) and spitting into a small glass vial for one to two minutes. Dr. Dabbs wryly observes that "chimps may take longer."

Popular belief about the relationship between testosterone and emotions and behavior has been limited to the correlation of higher levels of testosterone with violence and aggression. This gross correlation in no way does justice to the complex of issues involved in human emotion, behavior, and experience.

The results of Dr. Dabbs's studies include the following observations:

1. Testosterone levels cycle daily. They are highest in the morning, on awakening, and fall by as much as one-third to one-half throughout the day.
2. Testosterone levels rise and fall with experiences of success and failure in social encounters.

3. Sexual experience stimulates a rise in testosterone, more for women than for men.
4. In an initial study of ninety-two men in eight occupations and an unemployed category, ministers were lowest in testosterone, while professional football players and actors were highest.
5. Trial lawyers have higher levels of testosterone than nontrial lawyers.

An overview of Dr. Dabbs's research leads to the conclusion that men and women with relatively higher levels of testosterone have both the challenge and the opportunity to access more aggressive energy than do men and women with lower levels. Some have the internal and external resources that help them learn to integrate and channel this energy adaptively and constructively. Some have only limited resources. Some have far *too* little. Research results show, for example, that college students who have levels of testosterone in the higher range show no corresponding inclination to antisocial behavior, while groups of other "high testosterone" individuals lacking educational direction or some other focus or structure in their lives are more likely to demonstrate delinquency, substance abuse, and social instability.

Dr. Dabbs stresses that "to understand human nature, it is imperative to understand both biologic and social forces." He adds that "behavioral or biological approaches alone are incomplete." His work proves that "testosterone affects behavior, but the outcome of behavior also affects testosterone levels."

Some women who have been accustomed to having a relatively high level of testosterone and who experience a radical drop at peri-menopause or menopause (or with hysterectomy or chemotherapy) may find the loss of vital energy more disturbing than women whose baseline levels of testosterone throughout their adult lives have been relatively lower. Parallel reasoning holds for men whose testosterone diminishes with aging.

"How can I get a measurement of saliva testosterone?"

I know of one commercial laboratory, Aeron Life Cycles, in San Leandro, California, that performs the assay and will provide materials for saliva collection and mailing.

Many physicians who treat women for symptoms of testosterone deficiency do not regularly order a blood test to measure their testosterone levels. Most have never even heard of the saliva test. Even my present gynecologist is fond of saying, "I treat the patient, not the numbers." There is something to be said for this philosophy, as long as the physician knows what she or he is doing, and as long as the patient is knowledgeable and comfortable with the approach.

Speaking for myself, though, I preferred to know what my pre-treatment testosterone levels were, and I requested intermittent tests to monitor blood levels as I began to supplement testosterone. (I was not using methyltestosterone, so the tests gave useful readings.) The bottom line, where testing levels of testosterone is concerned, is to monitor testosterone levels during supplementation, in order to assure that testosterone remains within the physiological range.

❧ 6 ❧

"THE NATURAL WAY?"

TAKE CARE!

"I've always planned to get through menopause without hormones—you know, the natural way."

Have you ever thought about what your life might have been like without the benefits of science, technology, and Western medicine? When I think about "the natural way"—which these days seems to mean *without Western medicine*—I realize that I might have died at age six of a ruptured appendix, or at age twenty-five of a complication of German measles that temporarily interfered with my blood's ability to clot. Who knows how many other times I was protected from potentially fatal viral or bacterial infections by immunization or antibiotics?

The natural way, for me, was to develop testosterone deficiency at age forty-eight, the symptoms of which yielded not at all to the ministrations of the best homeopaths, Chinese herbalists, acupuncturists, and healers of eclectic persuasion I consulted over a period of several years. Although none of them helped, several of these adventures were unusual and interesting. Two were particularly unpleasant: an "aggravation" from one homeopathic remedy and a phototoxic reaction from an herbal poultice.

The natural way is not necessarily benign.

It's pretty clear that nature has not designed us to outlive our reproductive years. At the beginning of this century the average life expectancy was forty-seven. We owe it to the advances of science, technology, and medicine that today's fifty-year-old American or British woman statistically can expect to live to be eighty-one.

"Are there other ways to help libido and energy if I don't want to use hormones?"

I have no doubt that some women are helped through the use of herbs, homeopathy, acupuncture, and other conceivable nonhormonal methods to maintain a balance and quality of life that works for them. It stands to reason that the women who contact me are those who have not found a good enough alternative solution to a loss of libido and energy that is unacceptable to them.

What I know for sure is that I and many other women have tried mightily to find alternative help, and that for me and for them nothing but supplementary testosterone has been effective in restoring vital energy, sexual libido, sensation, and response.

In the words of one of the women who consulted me and who has tried alternative approaches:

After my herbal regime failed, I sought homeopathic care, and after one dose of pulsatilla followed by several doses of arsenicum, the hot flashes and anxiety attacks disappeared. Several months later, they came back full force. I might also mention that for the past ten years or so my libido has plummeted, I have lost at least fifty percent of my pubic hair, and have noticed an increasing loss of upper-body strength.

Many of us wish that we could find a solution to these symptoms without having to take hormones. Among the alternative approaches I tried before using supplementary testosterone was consultation with the master of Chinese herbs and acupuncture, Ted Kaptchuk, author of *The Web That Has No Weaver.* He worked patiently, carefully, respectfully, and earnestly on my behalf—and I was hopeful to the last. But when herbs and acupuncture did not prove fruitful, he was entirely supportive of my ultimate exploration of testosterone supplementation.

Homeopathy was another healing art I tried. In consultation with one of Boston's leading practitioners, I took the prescribed remedy and promptly developed such a severe and enduring agitation that I was both impressed with the power of homeopathy and very much disinclined to risk any further experience of it.

Susun Weed, author of *Wise Woman Ways for the Menopausal Years,* is considered by many to be an authority on the use of herbal remedies. In her book, she makes note of the decrease, and in some cases total loss, of sexual desire experienced by many women at midlife. Ms. Weed urges women to work to make peace with themselves through this transition. Her words are poetic and powerful:

> *You may think your sexual desire is waning, may fear it is leaving you. But observe patiently, my sweet. . . . If you will but hold your wise blood inside and stir it in your own cauldron, you will nourish your kundalini, your serpent power, and find yourself, at sixty, passionately sexual with all of life!*

This does sound wonderful. But the sixty-year-old women who have been consulting me mourning their continued lack of sexual desire are most definitely not enjoying fulfillment of any promise of natural sexual rejuvenation. I am sorry to report that I have found no epidemiological study to demonstrate a pattern of natural reclamation of lost libido by aging women.

Even though Ms. Weed counsels patience, she does offer some suggestions of herbs that might "increase your libido." She lists as potentially useful such plants as fenugreek, Jacob's groundsel, Oriental ginseng, and oatstraw. Having heard of some other herbs that might generate some of the effects of testosterone, I called Ms. Weed to ask her about them. She first insisted that I tell her something about how I came by my interest in this material, and soon had me telling the sad tale of my several years searching for alternative approaches to symptoms of testosterone deficiency.

As I spoke, I felt a little defensive and apologetic about having given up on herbs and having succumbed to the use of hormones. Ms. Weed spoke up clearly and said, "You *do* come to a point where taking a drug is the solution." She went on to explain that her approach to any health problem has seven possible steps, the first being "do nothing." Should the problem not resolve by itself, the next step is to "collect information." The following three steps involve the use of herbs to "engage the energy," "for nourishment," and, failing resolution of the problem, "for sedation or stimulation." If the problem persists, the next step is "use supplements" (vitamins and minerals) or drugs (including hormones). For problems that have resisted all prior efforts and where such treatment might be indicated, the last step in Ms. Weed's hierarchy is "break and enter"—her appellation for surgery or other invasive manipulation.

After listening to my story, Ms. Weed kindly affirmed that it was apparent I had made my way through the alternative steps and that using drugs was not something to be apologetic about or to resist. She did encourage me to try some infusions of oatstraw and stinging nettle as nourishment to support my hormone-dependent body. I've tried the oatstraw so far. It's very pleasant, and allegedly a good source of calcium. The nettle hasn't beckoned to me as yet.

"What's the difference between 'natural' progesterone and synthetic progesterone? Doesn't natural progesterone come from yams?"

Confusion exists in the idea that "natural" progesterone is found in wild Mexican yam root. In fact, the wild Mexican yam root of the genus *Dioscorea* is a rich source of chemicals known as diosgenins. They and other plant molecules, known as sapogenins, have a chemical makeup very close to the basic steroid structure from which human steroid hormones, including progesterone and cortisone, are made, but yam root does not contain progesterone, nor can progesterone be derived from yam root by means of any simple extraction process. A chemical synthesis is necessary to make progesterone from diosgenins. I have found no reliable source of information to demonstrate that humans can obtain progesterone effects directly from yam, soybean, or any other plant chemicals.

I have been disturbed to learn, from several reliable sources, that some "wild Mexican yam creams" that are sold in natural-food or health stores actually contain synthesized progesterone that has been added to the yam root extracts reported on the labels! No mention is made on the label about the added hormone, since the product could not then be sold without a prescription. The problem is, any woman using Mexican yam root cream spiked with progesterone cannot know how much of the hormone she may be using. One compounding pharmacist who sells this cream tells me that it is "common knowledge" that the concentration of added progesterone in this cream amounts to 3 percent. On the basis of this information, he has calculated that the "yam cream" contains thirty-five milligrams of added progesterone per one-quarter teaspoon.

If a woman using this product is also taking supplementary estrogen, depending upon how much of the yam cream she may be using and absorbing, there is the possibility that she may not be getting enough progesterone and consequently may be at greater risk for developing cancer of the uterus. Or she may be getting too much progesterone, with a confusion of possible effects.

Some women think that the diosgenins in yam root extract are more natural than the progesterone that is made from them. This is a misapprehension. Studies of the effects of plant estrogens (phytoestrogens) show that plant sterols can attach to human hormone receptors, but that the effects they create are not the same as the effects of human hormones that ordinarily act at these receptor sites. However, the progesterone made from plant sterols exactly replicates the hormone made in our bodies. Nothing could be more natural than that.

Before 1940, progesterone could only be obtained from the urine of pregnant pigs, at a cost of about thirty-five thousand dollars per pound of hormone. In 1939, a chemist, Russell E. Marker, developed a technique for synthesizing progesterone from plant diosgenins, at an eventual cost of about five dollars per pound of hormone! Marker went on to found Syntex Corporation, a pioneering producer of synthetic hormones, including the birth-control pill.

Today Upjohn Pharmaceuticals is the major producer in the United States of "natural" testosterone and progesterone. Upjohn technical development specialist Kenneth Ball describes Upjohn's products as "semisynthetic"—that is, they begin as natural, complex plant sterols (obtained from extracts of soybean byproducts) which are then modified chemically to produce formulas identical to the steroids produced by the human body. These hormones are natural in that they are identical, molecule for molecule, to the hormones produced by ovaries, adrenal glands, and other tissues. Neither Upjohn nor any other drug company whose products are listed in the *PDR* makes testosterone or progesterone capsules, pills, creams, or gels that can be prescribed by a doctor and used by a woman who needs the hormone. The only source of testosterone and progesterone preparations for women is a pharmacy that can obtain the hormone in bulk from Upjohn or an intermediary and make to order ("compound") the capsules, creams, or whatever else the doctor has prescribed.

Because progesterone and testosterone are molecules that appear in nature, they cannot be patented or "owned" by any pharmaceutical manufacturer. It seems obvious that there is a large economic incentive for drug companies to develop synthetic drugs whose actions are meant to duplicate (or, if possible, improve upon) the functions of the natural hormones *and whose formulas they can own*. And it is these proprietary drugs that the drug companies advertise, promote, and list in the *PDR*, a book published by a publisher aptly named Medical Economics. In short, progesterone and testosterone are not promoted by drug companies because the margin for profit is limited.

"How is natural progesterone better than the brand-name synthetics?"

First, I want to emphasize that the term "natural" progesterone is a redundancy. Progesterone is progesterone. A molecule of progesterone made by a pharmaceutical company is indistinguishable from a molecule of progesterone made by a woman's ovary. The compounds that are not natural are compounds that mimic some of the actions of progesterone, but are chemically different.

The term "progestin" applies to any formula that has progesterone-like action, including progesterone. This means that progesterone is a progestin, and although progesterone can be synthesized, other synthetic progestins exist that are not progesterone. The two most commonly prescribed progesterone mimics are known chemically as medroxyprogesterone acetate and norethindrone, and are found in the brand-name pharmaceuticals Provera, Cycrin, Amen, Aygestin, and Micronor.

Still, some confusing usage has crept in, because for a long time any progestin was sometimes referred to as progesterone. For example, Provera and Cycrin were referred to as progesterone. That's why many of us use the redundant term "natural progesterone" when we *mean* simply and only progesterone.

Like progesterone, the proprietary synthetic progestins in proper dosage will control the buildup of the lining of the uterus, protecting a woman who is also taking supplementary estrogen from added risk of cancer of the uterus. And yet a significant body of anecdotal data and some subsequent research has added weight to the emphatic message of the "natural progesterone" pioneer, Dr. Katharina Dalton, whose 1977 book, *The Premenstrual Syndrome and Progesterone Therapy*, emphasized the undesirable differences between proprietary progestins and natural progesterone. Almost thirty years ago, Dr. Dalton made the case that natural progesterone has beneficial effects that other progestins do not have, including her claim that natural progesterone can very significantly help premenstrual syndrome, while other progestins may actually make the symptoms worse.

Today, we also know that those synthetic progestins can work against the most desirable balance of cholesterol, even canceling some of the beneficial effects of supplementary estrogen. Thanks to the three-year PEPI study, though, we know that **natural progesterone does not cause undesirable changes in fat metabolism.**

In addition, some women find that the synthetic drugs cause bloating, depression, tension, and other very unpleasant-to-intolerable symptoms. Natural progesterone is better tolerated by many women, although some few women may not be able to take it because it makes them lightheaded or sleepy. As natural progesterone is used by the body, it breaks down to forms that have sedative properties. Some women develop higher levels of these sedative steroids than others. Sometimes this problem can be solved by adjusting the dose and taking the medication at bedtime.

One little-known and important consideration exists with regard to the choice of using natural testosterone versus methyltestosterone. As we discussed in Chapter 3, testosterone is a precursor of estrogen and can be acted upon by an enzyme (an "aromatase"), which converts it to estradiol (one form of estrogen).

Methyltestosterone is not readily aromatized to estradiol.

For women who have had cancer where it may be desirable to keep estrogen levels as low as possible while allowing for the benefits of testosterone supplementation, methyltestosterone may be the drug of choice. Even for women who have not had cancer and who use estrogen supplemental therapy to prevent heart attack, stroke, and osteoporosis, maintaining the lowest effective dose of estrogen may be prudent. For this reason, **methyltestosterone may actually be preferable to natural testosterone for long-term use.**

Men who take testosterone supplement and who use high doses of natural testosterone run the risk of developing very high blood levels of estradiol, which may be dangerous for older men who may already have arteriosclerotic changes in their blood vessels. High levels of estradiol in these circumstances have been associated with increased incidences of blood clots, heart attacks, and strokes.

Men using natural testosterone should be monitored to be sure that they do not develop undesirably high levels of estradiol.

For a long time, the major problem with natural progesterone (the same as with natural testosterone) was the fact that it was not well absorbed when taken orally. In 1977, Dr. Dalton used to treat her patients with progesterone by injection, by implants, and by suppository. The proprietary synthetic progestins were designed to be better absorbed from the stomach and intestines than progesterone.

The biggest advance both in natural progesterone and in natural testosterone therapy has been the development of different delivery systems, including creams that can be rubbed into the skin, sublingual tablets made specifically so that the hormone is taken up by the blood vessels under the tongue, and capsules of "micronized" natural progesterone or testosterone suspended in oil.

Micronization is simply a process of breaking up any substance into very fine particles. One of the large, telephone-accessible compounding pharmacies offers copies of a research paper proving that its particular formulation of micronized progesterone in oil is well absorbed. This pharmacy advertises that it has a "license" to produce this delivery system, which has been patented by the originators. Even though progesterone cannot be patented, manufacturers are scrambling to patent delivery systems for the hormone. Profits are the bottom line.

The PEPI study reported that the group of women taking "micronized natural progesterone" in a dose of 200 milligrams per day absorbed enough of it to provide adequate protection against uterine cancer and, in addition, demonstrated no interference with the blood-cholesterol benefits of estrogen.

Dr. Irma Mebane-Sims, program administrator of the PEPI study, underlined the fact that different formulations of micronized progesterone could have different absorptions. Adequate absorption is potentially important for establishing a good enough blood level of progesterone to have its desired effects on the lining of the uterus. When I remarked to Dr.

Mebane-Sims that the PEPI report does not specify whether the micronized progesterone they used was suspended in oil, she confirmed that the most favorable results in the PEPI study had been in the group of women receiving micronized progesterone in oil, but added that the details were "proprietary" to the drug company that had provided the formulation. Schering-Plough obtained a patent for their delivery system, and the new pharmaceutical, Prometrium, marketed by Solvay Pharmaceuticals, was launched in May 1998.

Until recently, doctors had preferred to prescribe brand-name synthetic progestins. The drugs were better absorbed than natural progesterone. The *PDR* was nice and clear. The drug salesmen were articulate. The samples were free. All drugstores carried the products. In addition, other doctors prescribe synthetic progestins and have done so for many years—which would afford some defense in case of a lawsuit with medical/legal questions as to whether a doctor is practicing standard medicine.

Once the results of the PEPI study were published, many women began asking their doctors about natural progesterone and more doctors have been learning to prescribe it and to help their patients find compounding pharmacies where they can get their prescriptions filled. Now that Prometrium, a pharmaceutical preparation of natural progesterone, is available, doctors have a fully comfortable choice. I look forward to the day when a proper pharmaceutical preparation of testosterone suitable for supplementation in women becomes a comfortable option for doctors as well.

"My grandmother used to tell me about a clinic in Europe where you could go for a 'rest cure' and some kind of special hormone injections. Was she on to something?"

Health spas (some rumored to be in Switzerland) that claimed (perhaps still do?) to rejuvenate aging men and women with injections of extracts taken from the glands of sheep or other mammals may indeed have been effective, to the extent that they were providing natural animal hormones, including testosterone, to their clients. But the "rejuvenation" would have lasted only as long as the treatments continued, and could yield no permanent benefit, since all hormonal effects are transient. Testosterone, for example, is cleared from the blood—taken up by receptors or excreted by the kidneys within one hour.

In addition, the use of fresh animal glandular material is potentially risky for many reasons. For one thing, the injection of foreign (nonhuman) protein can trigger a severe, possibly lethal, allergic reaction. *And* we know that hormones—from animal testes, ovaries, adrenal glands, and urine—are powerful agents that must not be dosed with disregard to the amounts given.

In the United States today, I know of no source of such fresh animal glandular material for injection, but I am alarmed at finding, readily available from "health" stores, products labeled as containing "bovine orchic substance." One such product has promotional material stating: "This extract comes from the testicles of *extremely* virile bulls." Since substantial amounts of testosterone taken orally can put a strain on the liver, and since the amount of testosterone in this "orchic substance" is not standardized and not even known, there may be some risk in using such a product. Natural remedies are sometimes classified as "herbals" or as "glandulars." It seems apparent that as long as a label reads "orchic substance," the product can be sold without a prescription, though should the label read "testosterone," it could not be sold over the counter.

Dr. Fredi Kronenberg, a researcher on menopause at Columbia University's College of Physicians and Surgeons, wrote a recent editorial in the journal *Menopause* entitled "Alternative Therapies: New Opportunities for Menopause Research," in which she observed that "most women assume that anything purchased in a natural food store not only is safe but also must be good for them."

No doubt this is an overstatement.

While few are as gullible as her statement implies, some men and women do use "natural" products without having all the facts, and may suffer potentially serious consequences if the products they use contain hormones. Hormones labeled as such and standardized for dosage and purity legally can be sold only by a registered pharmacy and only with a physician's prescription. At this time, I know of no dependably standardized source of animal testosterone.

One founder of a health-product line repeats the quite unlikely but engagingly glib statistic that "we now have more deaths from prescribed drugs than from organic disease." More than ever, with the glut of proprietary drugs (some wonderful and some somewhat dangerous) and the flood of natural herbs and formulas (again, some wonderful and some somewhat dangerous), we must take responsibility for ourselves and ask the important questions, collect the relevant information, and find the answers in order to decide what's good for us and what's not.

⚘ 7 ⚘

HORMONE REPLACEMENT THERAPY:
ESTROGEN, PROGESTERONE, *and*
TESTOSTERONE

"The important message that people need to get is that there is no clear right or wrong approach to hormone replacement, because we just don't have the research."
—Irma Mebane-Sims, Ph.D.,
program administrator for the PEPI study at the NIH

I believe that no matter how much research is done, there will probably *never* be a universal, comprehensive, "clear right or wrong approach to hormone replacement." Each woman is unique and presents the challenge of being her own long-term research study. What is clear to me is that taking the trouble to work with oneself and to find a doctor who can really help is worth the effort.

In a review of menopausal hormone therapy in the 1992 inaugural issue of the *Journal of Women's Health,* Dr. Trudy Bush, an epidemiologist at Johns Hopkins University, summarized: "The scientific evidence to date supports . . . the concept of hormonal therapy for use by most postmenopausal women . . . to maintain an active and full life."

People talk about hormone replacement therapy (HRT) as if it were a simple, complete answer to the problem of hormone depletion, but as much as we might wish, we cannot exactly reproduce the full, complex hormonal tapestry of our reproductive years. Having said that, though, with hormone *supplemental* therapy, we *can* provide our bodies with judicious amounts of estrogen and testosterone, to nourish and maintain the function of our tissues to the extent that aging allows. The unique role of supplemental testosterone for maintaining vital and sexual energy must challenge the automatic assumption that HRT means estrogen and progesterone. For many women, HRT means estrogen, progesterone, *and* testosterone.

Today, most women know that supplemental estrogen can be used to relieve the traditionally familiar symptoms of menopause, which include hot flashes, night sweats, genital dryness, genital atrophy, mood swings, memory fuzziness, and insomnia.

The two most important health reasons to consider using supplementary estrogen and progesterone are to protect our cardiovascular system and our bones.

Until menopause, women have statistically fewer heart attacks and strokes than men, due to the multiple cardioprotective effects of estrogen. At menopause, when the ovaries stop producing substantial estrogen, this protection that women have had is no longer available. After menopause, women and men have about the same levels of estrogen—and the same incidence of heart attacks and strokes. This statistic is worth repeating:

Studies show that postmenopausal women who take supplementary estrogen reduce their risk of heart attack and stroke by 50 percent.

Adding testosterone to the hormonal regimen can further benefit blood vessels and blood-clotting factors, but testosterone can sometimes lower HDL ("good cholesterol"). Healthy diet, exercise, and monitoring the lipid profile is a prudent balance in protecting a woman's cardiovascular system.

Supplementary estrogen is essential for many women to prevent osteoporosis. Most women know that adequate dietary calcium, vitamin D, and weight-bearing exercise are important contributors to the health of our bones. However, for women with a genetic tendency to develop osteoporosis, diet and exercise without supplementary estrogen have been shown *not* to be significantly effective. Adequate supplementary estrogen for these women can be crucial in maintaining their bone density.

Testosterone and progesterone have also been shown to contribute substantially to the maintenance of bones. Researchers in the Netherlands recently published their findings that progestins help to build bones by a different mechanism than estrogen, and consequently make an independent contribution to the prevention of osteoporosis. In addition, Dr. Joel Finkelstein and his coworkers at Massachusetts General Hospital in Boston have published several papers on their work with men whose bones were weakened as a result of testosterone deficiency caused by an unusual metabolic genetic condition, and reported that significant increases in bone density occurred when these men were treated with supplementary testosterone.

The Gallup survey sponsored by the North American Menopause Society found that while about one-third (34 percent) of the women polled reported that they were presently using HRT, more than half (58 percent) said they had never taken supplemental hormones. The remaining 8 percent had used HRT at some time in the past and had stopped. Given the array of potential benefits, it is important to consider why a woman might decide not to take supplemental estrogen at menopause. The survey reported that of women whose doctors had recommended HRT and who had chosen not to take it, 35 percent cited "side effects" as their reason. Dr. Klaiber, referred to in Chapter 5, emphasizes that, in his experience, too many women stop taking hormones because they are not comfortable with the progestin they are taking. His sadness and frustration comes through when he talks about women in their seventies who come into his office stooped and in pain from osteoporosis. The damage is done, and it is too late for much help.

"I take hormones for menopause. How long do I have to take them?"

The beneficial effects of estrogen (to protect bones and blood vessels and to maintain the health of genital tissues, for example) depend on taking it. If you stop the estrogen, you stop the benefit. If you have testosterone deficiency and are taking supplemental testosterone, stopping the testosterone will likewise stop the benefit. Of course, the same reasoning applies to the benefits of progestins.

The truth about side effects is that there is no substitute for patient and individual attention to the details of the way each woman's body responds to hormones. No routine schedule of HRT will work for every woman, but with experience, intelligence, flexibility, and care, a recipe for hormone replacement that both improves a woman's quality of life and protects her long-term health can be created.

No woman should settle for the alternative of HRT with miserable side effects or no HRT at all.

The Gallup survey showed also that "concerns over cancer" was the reason given by 26 percent of the women who chose not to take HRT. Unfortunately, cancer of the uterine lining (the endometrium) can and does develop even in women who have *never* taken hormone supplements. Enough research has been done to show that women who have a uterus and use supplementary estrogen are at somewhat greater risk for developing endometrial cancer, and that **the use of adequate progestin can entirely eliminate this**

additional risk. Just how much progestin constitutes "adequate progestin," though, is up for debate. One extreme in the spectrum of recommendations is represented by the opinion of Dr. R. Don Gambrell, Jr., professor of endocrinology and ob/gyn at the Medical College of Georgia, who advises a regular thirteen-day course of a progestin each month.

Research has shown that those women who go through menopause with few difficulties—whose bodies may produce adequate estrogen even after menopause—are actually at greater risk to develop endometrial cancer than postmenopausal women who take estrogen *and progesterone* supplemental therapy. In other words: **Women with a uterus who do not take HRT because they feel that they "do not need it" have a greater incidence of endometrial cancer than women who take estrogen and progesterone.**

Dr. Gambrell recommends something he calls the Progesterone Challenge Test, or PCT, even for women who are not using HRT. The PCT, a once-a-year procedure, involves giving a woman who is past menopause (even if she is not using estrogen) an injection of depot progesterone or a twelve-day course of oral progesterone, which, in the event of significant endometrial buildup, causes the lining of the uterus to shed. For these women, whose bleeding indicates that the uterine lining has been receiving estrogen stimulation, Dr. Gambrell recommends continued monthly dosing with a twelve-day course of progesterone to prevent potentially risky buildup of the uterine lining. At any point when "withdrawal bleeding" no longer occurs, the monthly progesterone cycle can be stopped, and the PCT resumed once per year as a preventative and check for endometrial cancer (the same course of action that would be recommended for those women who didn't show any withdrawal bleeding in the first place). Dr. Gambrell points out that women who have endometrial cancer will virtually always show withdrawal bleeding when given the PCT.

At the other end of the spectrum of recommendations for adequate progestin therapy—and of potential importance to women who have unpleasant side effects from the use of *any* progestin—are schedules of progestin to be taken for ten days every three months. When I discussed progestin therapy schedules with one clinical researcher, specifically the concept of progestin cycling (ten to twelve days of progestin out of twenty-eight), she responded with the colorful expression "Somebody pulled that idea out of their ear!"

The truth is that there is no precise scientific basis for any progestin schedule. A woman and her doctor can work out a modified schedule, and provided she immediately reports any unusual bleeding and has a yearly endometrial biopsy, she is going a long way toward protecting herself from added risk of endometrial cancer.

In considering the effects of including testosterone in a supplemental hormone regimen, it is useful to remember that testosterone is a precursor for estrogen. (Dr. Greenblatt, the pioneer clinician in testosterone use for women, suggested that testosterone can, in fact, be considered "a weak estrogen.")

Dr. Morrie Gelfand, professor of ob/gyn at McGill University in Montreal, along with his colleagues Drs. Alex Ferenczy and Christine Bergeron from the Department of Ob/Gyn at the Jewish General Hospital, conclude that "the presently available data support the concept that [the combination of] estrogen-androgen act on the endometrium in the same way as estrogens alone." Moreover, in a group of women taking only supplemental testosterone, Dr. Gambrell discovered no instances of endometrial cancer.

A woman with an intact uterus who uses both supplementary estrogen and testosterone must take the same responsible steps as a woman using estrogen alone to develop a regimen of adequate progestin and to be examined regularly by her doctor to avoid additional risk of endometrial cancer.

A clinician with thirty years' experience in treating women with supplementary estrogen, progestin, and testosterone, Dr. Gelfand recommends the equivalent of a dose of 10 milligrams of the progestin medroxyprogestrone acetate (Provera or Cycrin) for fourteen days per month to eliminate the possibility of overgrowth of the lining of the uterus. The PEPI study showed that natural micronized progesterone capsules in an oil suspension at a dosage of 200 milligrams per day were adequate to protect the lining of the uterus.

Results of research designed to test the potential *benefit* of testosterone for women with breast cancer were reported in 1987 in the *European Journal of Surgical Oncology*. This project, which was initiated almost thirty years ago in London by Dr. Irene Karydas and her coworkers, randomized a group of one hundred and fifty women diagnosed with breast cancer who, after being treated by mastectomy, received either no additional treatment or were treated with supplementary testosterone. The introduction to this research explains the rationale behind their decision to use testosterone for this group of women: "The administration of androgens such as testosterone . . . may produce remissions in premenopausal patients with advanced breast cancer, and before the advent of tamoxifen this was standard treatment in patients who were just postmenopausal."

Four years into the study, 75 percent of the women who had had cancer in their lymph nodes and were subsequently treated with testosterone were alive, as compared with only 37 percent of the women with similar severity of cancer who had not received testosterone. About 50 percent of each of the treated and untreated groups survived the twenty years. The twenty-year follow-up analysis of the research data showed that while testosterone treatment appeared to have short-term benefits, it was ultimately neither beneficial nor harmful to the women who received it.

While testosterone is not a cure for breast cancer, neither

does it appear to stimulate growth of breast cancer. In fact, testosterone is known to reduce the growth of cells lining the ducts in breast tissue, possibly reducing the risk for developing breast cancer in the first place.

In 1995, statistics show that one in eight or nine women will, at some point, develop breast cancer, making it a threat to every woman. In the PEPI study, the three-year trial of estrogen and progesterone demonstrated no increased incidence of cancer of the breast or uterus in women using hormones when compared with women not taking any hormones. A variety of causes other than hormones are implicated in many cancers.

As recently as June/July 1995, two more research papers have been published presenting conflicting data and conclusions with regard to the risk of breast cancer in postmenopausal women who take estrogen and progesterone.

The April 1994 review by the Committee on Gynecologic Practice distributed to patients at Massachusetts General Hospital and entitled "Estrogen Replacement Therapy for Women with Previously Treated Breast Cancer" states: **"More than fifty epidemiologic studies have failed to demonstrate consistently or conclusively a detrimental impact of replacement [supplementary] estrogen use on the incidence of breast cancer."**

This paper concludes:

No woman can be guaranteed protection from recurrence. The short-term and potential long-term benefits of ERT (estrogen replacement therapy) are well recognized and contribute to the quality and quantity of life in postmenopausal women. In postmenopausal women with previously treated breast cancer, consideration of ERT is an option but must be viewed with caution. Any possible benefit must be balanced by a thorough explanation of current knowledge which, by necessity, will entail consultation with the patient's oncologist. The uncertainty of this dilemma demonstrates that extensive randomized, prospective trials need to be performed in order to provide women with a rational and reasonable basis for therapeutic alternatives.

To me, this sounds like gobbledygook. However many "randomized, prospective trials" may ever be performed, until we have found a cure for breast cancer, we all live in dread.

In spite of the unsettled questions of risk and benefit, the use of testosterone for problems of libido following chemotherapy for cancer has been mentioned increasingly in the media. A recent article by Jane Brody in the *New York Times* notes that "those [women treated for cancer] suffering from a loss of sexual desire often respond well to treatment with low doses of testosterone, the libido hormone in both men and women."

Statistics are calculated by evaluating groups of women. Each one of us has her own individual and personal risk/benefit factors—genetic, constitutional, medical, historical, environmental, psychological, and spiritual—to figure into her own decision making. When I was forty-eight, felt flat and dead, not like myself at all, I searched, learned, and considered the options, risks, and benefits. I decided. Every day I live that decision with the peace of mind that I can have only by knowing and accepting that I am making the best choice I can for myself, all things considered. I am glad to be alive and feel like myself again. I am glad to be alive.

8

HOW TO SUPPLEMENT
TESTOSTERONE AND OTHER NEW
AND IMPORTANT INFORMATION

When, in 1991, I wanted to find information about available sources of testosterone, I went right to the obvious source, the *PDR*.

There was not one preparation of testosterone listed as a supplement for women suffering testosterone deficiency.

Four years later—in 1995—the only *PDR* listing for a testosterone supplemental preparation was a scrotal skin patch for men, which specified in its "contraindications" the warning that this dosage "must not be used in women." In 1997, a second pharmaceutical product became available *for men*. A transdermal skin patch, Androderm, for "intact non-scrotal skin, such as the back, abdomen, thighs, upper arms," was developed by TheraTech, Inc., a Salt Lake City company that specializes in the development and manufacture of innovative, controlled-release drug delivery technologies, systems, and products.

Androderm, a pharmaceutical marketed by SmithKline Beecham, is designed to provide physiological dosages of testosterone for men. As noted in the *PDR*, "Daily application of Androderm at approximately 10 P.M. results in a serum testosterone profile that mimics the normal circadian variation observed in healthy young men. Maximum concentrations occur in the early morning hours, with minimum concentrations in the evening."

As this book goes to press, Unimed Pharmaceuticals of Chicago is about to file a new drug application for Androgel—for men. Androgel is a natural testosterone USP in a colorless gel for direct application to the skin. Communication with Unimed indicates that men can look forward to the availability of Androgel the first of the new millenium.

Finally, in 1999, I can report that a testosterone skin patch *designed for women* and developed by TheraTech is being evaluated in ongoing, multicenter clinical trials. The funding and ongoing research and development of the testosterone patch for women, as well as its eventual marketing, is a project of Procter & Gamble Pharmaceuticals, who look forward to the prospect of its availability within the next two or three years.

But what about today? Today, the *PDR* lists one pharmaceutical preparation, Estratest, that includes testosterone and is approved for use "for women." The use of Estratest as a testosterone supplement for women suffering symptoms of testosterone deficiency is an example of "off-label use" of an FDA-approved pharmaceutical. "Off-label use" means the use of a pharmaceutical in a dosage other than specified or for treatment of a condition other than specified in the FDA-approved description on the label and in the *PDR*.

When you read what the *PDR* has to say about "indications for usage" for Estratest, you won't find any mention of testosterone deficiency. What you will find is that this drug has been manufactured and approved **"for treatment of moderate to severe vasomotor symptoms associated with menopause in those patients not improved by estrogens alone."** In other words, Estratest actually was developed and is still marketed *not* for testosterone deficiency, but as a short-term treatment for hot flashes that estrogen alone won't help.

The fact that a given pharmaceutical has been demonstrated to be safe enough and effective enough to meet FDA standards is a good baseline for its use. However, many pharmaceuticals have been found to be useful, and are regularly prescribed, in dosages and for conditions other than those specified on the label. A confounding reality is that Estratest is being used off-label as a testosterone supplement for women, but the FDA has yet to pass approval on a pharmaceutical preparation for women *for the purpose of testosterone supplementation and in physiological dosage.*

When a pharmaceutical company wants to develop, manufacture, and market a new product, such as a much-needed pharmaceutical preparation of testosterone in dosage optimal for women, for each potential product the drug company has to take out a New Drug Application (NDA) with the Food and Drug Administration (FDA), and with the FDA agree on the proposed drug's "indications for usage." The manufacturer then has to prove to the FDA, via research and clinical trials, that the given dosage of the proposed drug is both safe and effective with regard to the proposed indications for usage.

On first consideration, this sounds fine. Of course we want our federal agency to make sure that drug companies make safe and effective drugs. In its practice of protecting the public, though, there are confounding inconsistencies, with potentially serious consequences, in the FDA's function. One impressive glitch is the over-the-counter availability, in any health-food store or other retail display—alongside the vitamins—of the potent adrenal cortical hormone DHEA (dehydroepiandrosterone). As we have discussed (page 51), knowledge about the efficacy and safety of this "mother steroid" is rudimentary and limited, yet DHEA is freely available to anyone without a doctor's prescription.

Consistent policy would allow testosterone, estrogen, progesterone, thyroid hormone—any "natural" hormone for use without injection—to be sold as freely as is DHEA. Alternatively, conservatively, and consistently, DHEA belongs properly classified as a prescription drug, available only on prescription.

When I was doing my initial exploration into available testosterone preparations, I called one of Boston's leading gynecologists and experts in menopause, who recommended Estratest, stressing that I should "be sure to use the half-strength." What this implied to me was that some physicians, not knowing any better, prescribe Estratest full strength!

Manufactured and marketed since 1981, Estratest H.S. (for "**H**alf **S**trength") is a cumbersome combination of a fixed (and higher than useful or necessary for many women) dose (1.25 milligrams) of methyltestosterone and a fixed dose (.625 milligram) of estrogen. Most women need a lower dosage of testosterone, as well as independent and flexible dosing of estrogen. Estratest (full strength) is a pharmaceutical with 2.5 milligrams of methyltestosterone in combination with 1.25 milligrams of estrogen—four to eight times more testosterone than can help most women, and enough to potentially compound their misery.

Methyltestosterone taken orally for absorption via the stomach and intestines goes directly to the liver. It has been known for many years that the regular use of high doses of methyltestosterone taken orally can place a strain on the function of the liver and can cause liver damage. Just what may constitute a "higher dose," though, is not certain. A 1995 study showed that women who took an oral dose of 2.5 milligrams of methyltestosterone per day for two years showed no undesirable effect on liver function. Reports in the literature have shown that men who took methyltestosterone in oral dosages of 20 milligrams to 150 milligrams per day, however, developed serious liver pathology. Knowledge of the potential risk to the liver is more important for men using supplemental testosterone than for women, who would not properly be prescribed oral methyltestosterone in the higher dosage range.

The *PDR* lists pharmaceutical preparations of methyltestosterone, 10 milligram dosage—whose indications for usage are as a hormone supplement for men or for use in women "for the treatment of advancing inoperable (skeletal) breast cancer." In other words, large oral doses (potentially toxic to the liver) of methyltestosterone are prescribed by some oncologists for some women with bone metastases of advanced breast cancer. These drugs are not for hormone supplementation for women, and really should not be used by men, either, who would be better off with "the patch" insofar as the health of their liver is concerned.

I have discovered that there is a sensitive "window" of dosage that works best for a woman using supplemental testosterone. If she is taking more than she needs, she may not experience improvement in her libido and will feel worse— agitated, very hungry for food, and even depressed. Several women who consulted with me had "tried Estratest" and "didn't like it." This experience discouraged them and led them to conclude that supplemental testosterone "could not help." After trying a much lower dose (one-quarter to one-half the dose of Estratest H.S.), sometimes shifting to topical genital application, many of these women subsequently felt very comfortable and had real improvement of their symptoms.

Back in 1991, what was I to do? I remembered an article by Dr. Greenblatt, who pioneered the use of testosterone for women and who at one point suggested that "one quarter of a teaspoonful of a 1 percent testosterone cream applied locally to the genital area may be used to advantage." (His formula was compounded before the advent of "absorption enhancers," about which we will speak later.) I decided to try this. But where could I get it? This challenge introduced me to the network of compounding pharmacists who are, at this time, the only source of flexibly dosed natural or synthetic hormone preparations of testosterone in the United States.

Compounding pharmacies obtain the testosterone products they use in formulating their preparations from suppliers like The Upjohn Company, which manufactures testosterone cypionate and testosterone enanthate (which can be used for injection), testosterone propionate (which can be mixed as a gel or cream) and methyltestosterone (which can be taken orally)—all formulations of testosterone linked to other chemical elements that are designed to regulate its absorption via the various "routes of delivery." Upjohn also produces (and has produced for years) plain testosterone USP (in United States Pharmacopoeia Standards of Purity), which can be formulated by a compounding pharmacist in any dosage prescribed by a physician into any form requested.

"Why are pharmacies allowed to make formulations of hormones when pharmaceutical companies cannot?"

Since 1938, when the Food, Drug and Cosmetics Act was passed, pharmaceutical companies have been required to file New Drug Applications and to satisfy all requirements of proof of efficacy and safety for each formulation of a drug that they manufacture. When this law was passed, an exception was made for "repackagers" and "compounders," which allows licensed pharmacies to make individual prescriptions formulated to order on prescription of a physician.

Compounding pharmacies are strictly prohibited from "manufacturing" (making and storing in large quantity) their formulated pills, creams, and other preparations. They are also required to use only ingredients that "comply with the standards of an applicable United States Pharmacopoeia or National Formulary monograph."

Significantly stimulated by the call for hormone preparations, compounding has been on the upswing over the last decade, during which a legislative bill known as the Pharmacy Compounding Preservation Act (HR 598), sponsored by Rep. William Brewster (a licensed pharmacist no longer in practice), was presented before Congress. As its title implies, the purpose of the bill was to further clarify the exemption of 1938 and to "make the language stronger to leave no doubt that pharmacies have the right to compound drugs." The bill, with provisions and injunctions, was passed and signed in November 1997 and went into effect on November 1, 1998.

The compounding pharmacy I located in Boston (and, in fact, Boston has several) is one of several hundred such independent pharmacies in the United States whose pharmacists are known as "serious compounders"—licensed pharmacists who make up the sixty-two thousand prescriptions compounded to order each day.

In the course of my research on the subject of compounding, the name of one pharmacist, George Roentsch, of Keene, New Hampshire, came up repeatedly. When I asked my pharmacist, Steve Grossman, of Pierce Apothecary in Brookline, Massachusetts, if he had heard of Mr. Roentsch, Steve said, "George? He's incredible!"

Several telephone conversations with George supplied everything I could have wanted to know about compounding. He told me that he had always been interested in compounding, and that when he graduated from pharmacy school in 1957, some compounding was part of the regular practice of pharmacy. However, pharmaceutical drugs increasingly took over, until by the late sixties and early seventies, suppliers began to discontinue supplies of the raw materials needed for compounding.

By 1980, matters had come to a critical pass, at which point five pharmacists from Florida and Texas formed a group to buy the very expensive bulk supplies and to repackage the stock for distribution to compounding pharmacies. Eventually, they began to offer classes (which meet in Houston, Texas) to teach the newer compounding techniques to those licensed pharmacists who want to keep up with them. In 1991, a nonprofit group now known as the International Academy of Compounding Pharmacists, the IACP, was founded. Based in Houston, the group staffs an information hotline about compounding and compounding pharmacists.

In 1993, George Roentsch established, for the purpose of networking with other "serious compounders," the Pitcher

Mountain Electronic Bulletin Board Service. Members exchange information about all aspects of compounding, including anecdotal information about experiences with the needs of individual patients/clients and creative solutions they have worked out with the patients and prescribing physicians. George is very selective about his standards for membership. At present he has accepted 450 compounding pharmacists as qualified to use the service, nearly three times the number registered in 1995.

"Who oversees the compounding pharmacies?"

All licensed pharmacies come under the jurisdiction of each individual state's Board of Pharmacy. These authorities make regular inspections, check compounding logs, and oversee storage facilities for stocks of compounded drugs. Back in the olden days, before the era of proprietary pharmaceuticals, pharmacists regularly compounded prescriptions to order. Watching the disappearance of the independent drugstores in my hometown, I expected to find statistics to show that the small, neighborhood pharmacy was just about extinct. In 1995, I was pleasantly surprised to learn that, according to the figures of the National Association of Retail Druggists, independent "corner drugstores" still outnumbered the chain pharmacies twenty-eight thousand to twenty-three thousand. (Chains are considered to consist of four or more pharmacies.) Since there are additionally fourteen thousand or so hospital and clinic pharmacies, the total number of retail pharmacies in the United States is about sixty-five thousand. Three years later, in 1998, the numbers are, sadly, reversing somewhat. There are now twenty thousand independent pharmacies and thirty thousand chain pharmacies—a significant loss of corner drugstores.

Chain pharmacies, for the most part, do little compounding. Today, not many independent pharmacies do, either. Most pharmacies limit themselves to dispensing pharmaceuticals—drugs that have been manufactured and often already packaged by drug companies. Of the sixty-five thousand pharmacies in the United States, only about *twenty-five hundred* prepare compounded drugs to prescription. Nonetheless, that number is **up** significantly from the fifteen hundred compounding pharmacies that existed in 1995.

One competent gynecologist I know prescribes Estratest H.S. as a supplement for her patients who need and want to take testosterone. Both she and an endocrinologist I know direct their patients to cut the tablet into four pieces and to take one tiny bit each day.

Why do these doctors resist writing a prescription for a pharmacist to compound testosterone in a dose individualized to the patient's hormonal needs? One consideration is the fact that a doctor's confidence in the competence of a compounding pharmacist develops and grows as a result of the development of a working relationship between the physician and the pharmacist—and that is a matter of propinquity, chemistry (of the personal variety), and time. Another and daunting reality is the circumstance of physicians who work for managed care organizations and whose patients must obtain their medications from pharmacies that do not do compounding.

"I'm thirty-two, and I've heard about 'testosterone cream' on a TV show. I could use a boost to my sex drive. What about it?"

The short answer is: **If you can get pregnant, you MUST NOT USE TESTOSTERONE.** If a woman *of childbearing age* uses supplemental testosterone and happens to get pregnant, the testosterone can lead to disastrous consequences for the developing fetus. As we saw earlier (page 41) all fetuses begin development *as females*. Early in development, a surge of testosterone triggered by the presence of a single gene directs the subsequent sexual development of a male baby. If you are pregnant with a female baby, supplemental testosterone could cause serious developmental problems with her reproductive organs as well as in the "programming" of her sexual identity, including her brain.

The responsible use of physiological dosage of supplemental testosterone can be crucial to the maintenance of a woman's health and quality of life. It is not responsible to advise "younger women"—women of childbearing age—to "find a doctor who will give them testosterone cream." Women need to know the risks should they get pregnant.

"I'm past menopause, and I can't wait to try that '2 percent testosterone cream' I heard about on TV."

An old-fashioned remedy for topical testosterone was 1 percent or 2 percent testosterone in "petrolatum"—Vaseline. Today, chemists have designed "absorption enhancers"—chemicals that help the absorption of large molecules through the skin and into the blood. Absorption enhancers are used not only in pharmaceutical preparations, but also in cosmetics.

As much as we might wish to have one, today there is no single controlled pharmaceutical preparation of "testosterone cream." Since any topical preparation of testosterone can be formulated by any compounding pharmacy using any formula for a cream base, the composition of the cream base, including the effectiveness of the absorption enhancers used, will result in potentially widely different absorbencies of the same percentage concentration of testosterone.

Regular use of 2 percent testosterone on the genitals can result in excessive absorption of testosterone into the general circulation.

A woman who regularly uses 2 percent testosterone cream prepared with absorption enhancers is running an irresponsible risk of developing abnormally high blood levels of testosterone, with the unnecessary and undesirable potential "virilizing side effects": increased facial hair, acne, lowered voice, enlargement of the clitoris.

A significant amount of testosterone propionate is converted in the body to estrogen. Women who are at risk for development or recurrence of breast cancer or ovarian cancer and whose physicians advise keeping estrogen levels down need to know that **the regular use of 2 percent testosterone cream on the genitals can result in high blood levels of testosterone, some of which will be converted in their body to estrogen.**

TOPICAL TESTOSTERONE
FOR GENITAL USE

Having been consulted by hundreds of women, I have found that the most effective way to begin supplementation of testosterone is initially to apply it directly to the genital tissue. The key issue in this method is to **avoid overdosage.** A standardized pharmaceutical preparation for topical genital use is critically needed, since the absorption of the drug will vary according to the composition of the base prepared by the formulating pharmacy. The best we can do at present is to monitor both the clinical results and the blood levels of testosterone, in order to be sure that blood levels do not get above the normal range. Your doctor needs to familiarize him/herself with the "absorption profile" of the particular cream base used by the pharmacy making the testosterone cream. My experience is based on a cream prepared to my order by George Roentsch, of The Apothecary in Keene, New Hampshire. Another compounding pharmacy, Apothecare in Greenville, South Carolina, has formulated the same base for me.

The following concentrations and dosages are based upon my experience of women using these topical preparations.

Testosterone propionate USP, micronized natural testosterone USP, or methyltestosterone USP in a cream base with absorption enhancers —typically 0.25 percent or 0.5 percent and used in a dosage of 0.1-0.2 milliliters total per day.

This preparation of testosterone powder mixed with a cream base in the prescribed concentration is designed to be applied directly to the genital tissue. It can be used daily, after bathing, and should be used in tiny, carefully measured and dispensed amounts—typically 0.1–0.2 milliliter per day. Testosterone cream can lose potency over time, and so is best prepared in small quantities. Topical application of testosterone is a particularly good way to begin for women who have lost pubic hair, whose genital tissue is atrophic in spite of taking estrogen, and/or who have not used any hormone supplement (estrogen or testosterone) in the recent past. If a woman's genital tissue is particularly thin and withered, it can take several weeks for the tissue to improve and to absorb the testosterone into the general circulation. Still, this can be a particularly gentle and gradual way for a woman's body to accustom itself to the hormone.

I have been consulted many times by women who have used oral testosterone supplement, experienced some benefit to their general energy, mood, and muscle tone, but have had little improvement in sexual libido. Shifting to the use of topical testosterone cream applied directly to their genital tissue has brought about increased sensitivity to sexual sensation, improved capacity for orgasm, and increased sexual libido.

Like all hormones, testosterone is cleared from the blood very quickly. It is excreted in the urine or metabolized by the liver and excreted in the bile within an hour. Another advantage of topical testosterone, then, is that it remains on the tissue, supplying the hormone over time. Especially at the outset, when testosterone receptors are depleted, to have testosterone supplied more continuously can be helpful.

As with topical estrogen, when testosterone is applied to less atrophic genital tissue, it can be very readily absorbed, potentially resulting in undesirably high blood levels. As with testosterone taken orally, testosterone absorbed topically can be metabolized to estradiol. Blood tests can be conducted periodically and the dosage and application adjusted to keep blood levels effective and within a normal range. I would be reluctant to maintain testosterone at levels above the normal range because of potential undesirable effects on the liver and on cardiovascular risk factors, as well as the potential of undesirable virilizing effects.

If topical testosterone is used long enough for spontaneous genital stimulation to occur, it is a signal to cut back the percent dosage and/or frequency of application. Increase in size of the clitoris could occur, though this is not a dramatic development that happens overnight. The topical preparation can be discontinued if any increase in size begins to occur. Minor increase is reversible on discontinuance of the topical testosterone. A shift to oral testosterone supplement would be indicated at this point.

A point that bears repeating: Women who are at particular risk for development or recurrence of breast cancer or ovarian cancer and whose physicians advise keeping estrogen levels down can use methyltestosterone in an absorption-enhanced cream base, which is least likely to convert in their body to estrogen. The use of methyltestosterone, however, confounds the blood test for testosterone—and care must be taken not to use the topical preparation longer than needed to "jump start" a response, at which point a shift to oral methyltestosterone would be advisable.

TESTOSTERONE CAPSULES
FOR ORAL USE

While some women like the idea of using a "natural" hormone over its synthetic derivative, the truth is that methyltestosterone is more readily absorbed when taken by mouth than is natural testosterone, so that a lower dosage can be effective. As we have seen earlier, methyltestosterone does not readily convert to estradiol, as does natural testosterone. For women, an appropriately low dose of testosterone taken by mouth would not likely raise the overall estrogen level to a significant degree.

The most effective oral dose of methyltestosterone ranges from .25 milligram to .75 milligram, with most women benefitting from a dose of about .5 milligram. Any higher, lower or intermediate dose can be prescribed and compounded. The one potential disadvantage is the fact that the blood test for testosterone is confounded in the presence of methyltestosterone. At the low dosages recommended, however, there is no risk of testosterone levels developing above the normal range—and so little reason to monitor them.

A useful dosage range for natural micronized testosterone is more variable, due both to the fact that it is less easily absorbed than methyltestosterone and that, once taken into the body, it is metabolized to other forms, including estradiol. The best course for each woman is to decide with her doctor which form of testosterone makes most sense to use, and then to begin at a lower dose of the hormone, watching for effects at that dose level for several weeks before adjusting the dosage upward.

In compounding the prescription, the pharmacist should use clear capsules, free of dyes, sugar, or sugar substitute, mixing the prescribed dose of testosterone with an inert base. **Women who are lactose intolerant should specify to the pharmacist *not* to use lactose.** (George Roentsch recommends methylcellulose as an excellent base). If a dose of .5 milligram of methyltestosterone is not effective within three weeks, it may be helpful to "jump start" the effects of testosterone by shifting to a few weeks' use of 0.25 percent or 0.5 precent testosterone cream, as described above.

TESTOSTERONE AND ZINC DEFICIENCY

A fascinating study published in 1996 jointly by physicians from Harvard Medical School and Wayne State University

School of Medicine in Detroit showed a correlation between zinc deficiency and serum testosterone levels in normal men. The researchers made the point that zinc deficiency is prevalent throughout the world, including the United States. Supplemental zinc, in a dosage of 15 milligrams to 30 milligrams, is a simple nutritional support for our general health and potentially to enhance our testosterone blood levels. It is important not to take more than 30 milligrams of zinc per day, since excessive zinc supplement can interfere with copper metabolism, with the risk of disturbing the balance needed for hemoglobin production and red blood cell health.

"And what about Viagra for women?"

I attended a recent meeting of leaders in the field of female sexual dysfunction, where preliminary anecdotal information was presented of research with some women who suffered loss of libido following hysterectomy. Angiograms showed the reduced blood supply to the pelvis that resulted from the surgery—as well as the increased blood supply apparent when women taking Viagra were sexually stimulated. It makes sense to me that increased blood supply to the pelvis can enhance sexual response for some women, particularly if they are suffering from injury to the blood supply as a consequence of surgery.

My own collection of anecdotal data, gathered from colleagues who have prescribed Viagra "off-label" to women urging to be allowed to try it, as well as from a woman who is herself a physician (whose husband gave her one of his pills on her fifty-sixth birthday) shows mixed results. A few women reportedly noticed some enhancement of sexual feeling. The menopausal woman-physician noticed no effect whatsoever, and has elected to re-regulate her testosterone and estrogen supplement.

*"Is the medical community becoming more receptive
to providing supplemental testosterone to women
who can benefit from it?"*

Somewhat. However, even in June 1998, the distortions
that are sometimes presented to discourage physicians from
prescribing testosterone and to frighten women about taking
it are impressive. At that recent conference on female sexual
dysfunction, one speaker elected to present a talk focused on
signs and symptoms of testosterone **excess** in women, illus-
trated by a display of slides—photos of teenage girls with severe acne and excessive facial and body hair, and middle-aged
women balding at the top of the head. In his remarks, the
speaker chose to emphasize how distressed women are about
losing their hair.

No question about it—women do not want to go bald!!
And those women whose hair thins and falls out with aging are
unfortunately losing their hair **not** because they have too
much testosterone, but because they are genetically programmed to lose their hair.

For sure, news about the role of testosterone in normal female physiology is making its way into the popular press. On
February 24, 1998, Jane E. Brody's column in *The New York
Times* was entitled, "A Tad of Testosterone Adds Zest to
Menopause"—and it has been excerpted in the July 1998
issue of *Readers' Digest* with the title "Do You Need the 'Hormone of Desire'?"

TESTOSTERONE, HYSTERECTOMY, AND
CARDIOVASCULAR HEALTH

A recent publication in *The British Medical Journal* reports that as women age our incidence of risk factors for coronary heart disease and death equals that of men. In 1997, the
Rancho Bernardo Study was published, confirming what
other studies had shown before, which was that removal of the

ovaries, *even in women who received estrogen supplemental therapy after the surgery,* resulted in **increased heart disease risk factors.**

A series of publications over the past twenty years has shown that women who have had a hysterectomy have three to seven times the risk of heart attack and stroke compared to women who have not had the surgery—even if their ovaries have been left in place, and even if they have been treated with supplementary estrogen.

Common ignorance has implicated testosterone as the reason why men have more and earlier heart attacks than women. It seems evident to me that men have greater cardiovascular risk *not* because they have testosterone, but because they *don't have estrogen.* In fact, as men age, not only do they live without the protection of estrogen, but they also experience some decrease in their potentially protective testosterone as well.

My paper, recently published in *The Journal of Womens's Health,* points to testosterone deficiency as a significant factor contributing to the reported increased incidence of cardiovascular disease risk to women who have had a hysterectomy. We have seen (page 60) how, even if the ovaries are left in place at the time of hysterectomy, they can suffer damage—with the resulting loss of estrogen and of testosterone. We know that when the ovaries aren't functioning at their best, the adrenal cortices don't function fully, either—with a loss of that source of testosterone. **Too infrequently diagnosed are the consequences of the drop both in estrogen and in testosterone that can occur even for women whose ovaries have not been removed at the time of hysterectomy.** In light of the potential benefits to cardiovascular health, to bones, to sexuality, and to quality of life, the challenge exists for our researchers to evaluate the potential risks/benefits of physiological dosing of supplemental testosterone for women and for men.

A forty-five-year-old woman recently consulted me together with her husband. The couple loved each other and felt that their marriage was suffering because of the woman's lack of sexual desire. Not yet menopausal, she described her experience of making love as "no more pleasant than reading a book." Often tired, she would frequently simply stop the lovemaking as "not worth the trouble." It turned out that she needed both estrogen and testosterone supplementation. A recent follow-up call found her delighted with her present energy and intense pleasure in lovemaking.

In the words of another woman after using supplemental testosterone: "I have a libido again. I feel whole as a woman. I feel like I have a full life again." And in the words of her husband: "We are back to the foolishness, the making love, the courting, kind of like we were twenty years ago. It's great."

Of course, if the circumstances of a particular woman's life are stressful and difficult, no amount of testosterone will neutralize the pain, but an adequate amount of effective testosterone will help a woman be as strong and whole as possible, better equipping her to deal with life.

A final word: In spite of misconceptions, fears, or even wishes, the truth is that supplementary testosterone will not stimulate some extraordinary degree of sexual desire, though it can restore to a woman a level of sexual aliveness that's familiar to her. As most women age, even this level moderates naturally, as the function of their testosterone receptors declines with age. With the option of using supplementary testosterone, though, women have the choice of maintaining their ability to enjoy whatever sexuality and vigor may be natural to them well into older age.

In closing, I will affirm what has always been and still remains my personal practice, where tampering with the natural order is concerned: Do as little as you can and as much as you need, and no one knows better than you.

✌ Afterword ✍

In the spring of 1991, when the last alternative approach to my symptoms had failed and just before I decided to try using supplemental testosterone, I had the following dream:

On an island. A huge ocean wave crests above houses along the shoreline. "I am going to die." Unusually calm, I surrender. Floating and swimming facedown in ocean water. Sounds overhead. Helicopters. Rope ladders. Rescue. Spits of land. Many people standing. Reaching down. Pulling up to safety. Calm and busy. Just before I awaken, I hear a voice:

"YOU ARE NOT ALONE."

I have been graced both with this dream of great compassion and with its actualization at critical times during the years of my work leading to the publication of this book. I am not religious. As I study the confoundingly complex interrelationships of hormones, genetic factors, metabolic pathways, and neurotransmitters, I feel as though I must look away from the page I am reading, as though I am risking looking into the face of God.

S.R.
Chatham, Massachusetts

✎ Notes ✎

FOREWORD

p. 17 "I think particularly": S. Waxenberg, 1959.

p. 19 "The dean speaks": Marcus Kogel, M. D., Albert Einstein College of Medicine, New York, 1962.

CHAPTER ONE

p. 25 "beginning with the 1940s publications by the late Dr. Robert Greenblatt": R. B. Greenblatt, 1942 (both), 1943, 1950.

p. 25 "that groundbreaking paper": S. Waxenberg, 1959.

p. 25 "A woman's normal physiology includes": J. Veldhuis, 1991.

p. 25 "This critical amount": N. McCoy, 1991.

p. 25 "Supplementary testosterone can be a substantial help": G. A. Bachmann, 1993; L. Cardozo, 1984; M. M. Gelfand, 1992; R. B. Greenblatt, 1942 (both), 1943, 1950, 1985, 1987; H. S. Kaplan, 1992, 1993; J. Money, 1961; H. Persky, 1982; U. J. Salmon, 1943; R. Sands, 1995; B. B. Sherwin, 1985 (all), 1987, 1993; J. W. W. Studd, 1977; R. L. Young, 1993.

p. 25 "Only the use of irresponsibly high doses": M. M. Gelfand, 1992.

p. 26 "She did an endometrial biopsy": R. D. Gambrell, 1992.

p. 26 "which makes *less available*": M. Elias, 1992.

p. 26 "While menopause clinics in England": M. Brincat, 1984; H. G. Burger, 1984; L. Cardozo, 1984.

p. 26 "Some physicians in Canada": M. M. Gelfand, 1992; B. B. Sherwin, 1985 (all), 1987, 1988.

p. 27 "developed blood levels": M. Brincat, 1984; H. G. Burger, 1984; R. Sands, 1995.

p. 27 "I had read of a method": R. B. Greenblatt, 1987.

p. 28 "There can be as many differences": E. Cole, 1988.

p. 28 "together with factors of aging": T. Hallstrom, 1977; E. Pfeiffer, 1972; N. McCoy, 1991.

p. 28 "And some physicians approach": G. McBride, 1993.

CHAPTER TWO

p. 32 "Only five of the hundreds": J. Bancroft, 1981, 1983; J. Money, 1961; B. B. Sherwin, 1985 (third listing), 1987.

p. 32 "From Greer's book": G. Greer, 1992, p. 177.

p. 33 "women without a male partner": H. G. Burger, 1984.

p. 34 "without the use of supplementary estrogen": N. McCoy, 1991.

p. 34 "A Gallup survey": W. H. Utian, 1994.

p. 35 "The majority of women": W. H. Utian, 1994.

p. 37 "Discouraging and typically misleading": G. McBride, 1993.

p. 37 "Only if taken in excessive dosages": M. M. Gelfand, 1992; R. Sands, 1995.

p. 39 *decrease their risk of heart attacks*": R. A. Lobo, G. McBride, 1993; S. H. Ravn, 1994; Writing Group for the PEPI Trial, 1994.

p. 39 "women using adequate supplementary estrogen": J. C. Gallagher, 1993; R. Lindsay, 1991.

p. 39 "the results of a three-year study": Writing Group for the PEPI Trial, 1994.

CHAPTER THREE

p. 41 "testosterone plays the key role": H. S. Kaplan, 1993.

p. 42 "puberty for both girls and boys": R. M. Rose, 1972.

p. 42 "there is also an adrenopause": D. C. Cumming, 1982.

p. 42 "a woman's ovaries primarily produce": S. S. C. Yen, 1991.

p. 42 "Enough testosterone remains unconverted": C. Longcope, 1986.

p. 43 "adult males have": R. M. Rose, 1972.

p. 43 "there are testosterone receptors in the skin": R. B. Greenblatt, 1985; J. Money, 1961; S. E. Waxenberg, 1959.

p. 43 "there are testosterone receptors in the nipples": R. B. Greenblatt, 1985.

p. 43 "as well as in the clitoris": R. B. Greenblatt, 1943, 1985; J. Money, 1961; U. J. Salmon, 1943.

p. 43 "There are receptors *in the brain*": R. B. Greenblatt, 1943, 1985; B. S. McEwen, 1984, 1991; J. Money, 1961; U. J. Salmon, 1943.

p. 43 "only male canaries sing": R. B. Greenblatt, 1985.

p. 44 "Testosterone and other androgens": J. Veldhuis, 1991.

p. 44 "Without enough effective testosterone": G. A. Bachmann, 1993; R. B. Greenblatt, 1987; J. Veldhuis, 1991.

p. 44 "From the 'kickoff' of testosterone production": J. Veldhuis, 1991.

p. 44 "Testosterone is carried in the blood": S. S. C. Yen, 1991.

p. 45 "Estrogen actually stimulates the production of *more* SHBG": S. S. C. Yen, 1991.

p. 45 "testosterone works by attaching to": J. Veldhuis, 1991.

p. 45 "Sensitivity to testosterone is a variable": H. S. Kaplan, 1993.

p. 46 "By no means is it true": J. Money, 1961.

p. 46 "These symptoms of excessive testosterone use": R. Sands, 1995.

p. 47 "I have experienced a lag time": J. Bancroft, 1981, 1983; R. B. Greenblatt, 1950; K. A. Hutchinson, 1995.

p. 47 "Other effects of testosterone deficiency can include": J. A. Finkelstein, 1989.

p. 47 "loss of muscle tone in the bladder and pelvis": R. B. Greenblatt, 1942, 1987.

p. 47 "in conjunction with Kegel exercises": R. R. Freedman, 1994.

p. 48 "the degree of activity of a particular skin enzyme": J. Veldhuis, 1991.

p. 48 "Drs. Stein and Leventhal observed": I. F. Stein, 1935.

p. 48 "Dr. Yen explains that the onset": S. S. C. Yen, 1991.

p. 49 "Dr. Richard S. Legro": R. S. Legro, 1995.

p. 50 "Dr. Florence Haseltine has cautioned": F. P. Haseltine, 1995.

p. 51 "LSA is due to reduced activity of the same skin enzyme": E. G. Friedrich, Jr., 1984.

p. 51 " 'another adrenal androgen called DHEA' ": N. Orentreich, 1984.

p. 51 "showing the 'protective effects of DHEA' ": E. Barrett-Connor, 1986; P. Ebeling, 1994; S. S. C. Yen, 1991.

p. 52 "In 1994, Dr. Yen and his research associates reported": A. J. Morales, 1994.

p. 52 "consider DHEA to be the 'mother steroid' ": W. Regelson, 1994.

CHAPTER FOUR

p. 55 "during our mid- to late teens": N. Orentreich, 1984.

p. 56 "in order for a woman's adrenal glands to produce": D. C. Cumming, 1982.

p. 56 "While men's adrenal glands also show a drop": N. Orentreich, 1984.

p. 57 "for 50 percent of women, when the ovaries stop": C. Longcope, 1980.

p. 57 "a woman may experience some increase": H. L. Judd, 1974; B. B. Sherwin, 1987 (first listing), 1993.

p. 57 " 'When it occurs, this increase in ovarian testosterone production' ": B. B. Sherwin, 1993.

p. 58 "A gradual development of testosterone deficiency": C. Longcope, 1986; N. L. McCoy, 1991; E. Pfeiffer, 1972.

p. 58 "are likely to develop testosterone deficiency precipitously": S. Chakravarti, 1977; R. B. Greenblatt, 1976; B. B. Sherwin, 1985 (all), 1988.

p. 59 **"one-third of American women"**: V. Hufnagel, 1988; W. H. Utian, 1994.

p. 59 "She writes about the outrage": V. Hufnagel, 1988.

p. 61 **"can expect to go through menopause four years earlier"**: N. L. McCoy, 1991.

p. 61 "women whose ovaries are functionally wiped out": H. S. Kaplan, 1992.

CHAPTER FIVE

p. 65 "These expressions are echoed": E. Cole, 1988.

p. 66 "The hair-forming elements (PSU's, or 'pilosebaceous units')": R. L. Rosenfield, 1995.

p. 67 "the majority of healthy men": D. T. Villareal, 1994.

p. 68 "the Massachusetts Male Aging Study": H. A. Feldman, 1993; J. B. McKinlay, 1989, 1993, 1994.

p. 70 "And yet a few cautions exist": J. S. Tenover, D. T. Villareal, 1994.

p. 71 "the potential use of testosterone as an 'anabolic tonic' ": D. T. Villareal, 1994.

p. 72 "Researchers at Columbia Medical School reported": G. B. Phillips, 1994.

p. 73 "In an early study, published in 1946": M. A. Lesser, 1946.

p. 73 "the benefits of testosterone treatment of patients with occlusive vascular disease": G. R. Fearnley, 1962.

p. 73 "vital role of anabolic steroids in regulating blood sugar": M. L. Tainter, 1964.

p. 73 "men whose electrocardiogram showed evidence of": M. D. Jaffe, 1977.

p. 74 "The best-known and most commonly used method": A. Yamaguchi, 1988.

p. 77 "A laboratory method that utilizes saliva": J. M. Dabbs, Jr., 1990, 1991; J. Vittek, 1985.

p. 78 "To understand fully the relationships between hormones and behavior": J. M. Dabbs, Jr., 1993.

p. 78 "Testosterone levels cycle daily": Personal communication with Dr. Dabbs, 1995.

p. 79 " 'to understand human nature, it is imperative' ": J. M. Dabbs, Jr., 1993.

CHAPTER SIX

p. 83 "the master of Chinese herbs and acupuncture": T. Kaptchuk, 1984.

p. 83 "an authority on the use of herbal remedies": S. Weed, 1992.

p. 88 "the 'natural progesterone' pioneer": K. Dalton, 1977.

p. 88 "Thanks to the three-year PEPI study": Writing Group for the PEPI Trial, 1994.

p. 89 "As natural progesterone is used by the body": E. S. Arafat, 1988.

p. 89 "which may be dangerous for older men": E. L. Klaiber, 1982.

p. 90 "Micronization is simply a process": J. T. Hargrove, 1989.

p. 90 "Dr. Irma Mebane-Sims": Personal communication, 1995.

p. 92 "Testosterone, for example, is cleared from the blood": R. Sands, 1995.

p. 92 " 'most women assume that anything purchased' ": F. Kronenberg, 1995.

CHAPTER SEVEN

p. 94 " *The important message that people need* ": Personal communication, 1995.

p. 94 "In a review of menopausal hormone therapy": T. L. Bush, 1992.

p. 95 "The two most important health reasons": J. C. Gallagher, 1993; R. Lindsay, 1991; R. A. Lobo, 1993; G. McBride, 1993; S. H. Ravn, 1994; Writing Group for the PEPI Trial, 1994.

p. 95 "Adding testosterone to the hormonal regimen": H. G. Burger, 1984; M. M. Gelfand, 1992; B. B. Sherwin, 1987 (first listing).

p. 96 "for women with a genetic tendency to develop osteoporosis": R. Lindsay, 1991.

p. 96 "Researchers in the Netherlands": H. J. Verhaar, 1994.

p. 96 "Testosterone and progesterone have also been shown": J. S. Finkelstein, 1989; J. C. Prior, 1990.

p. 96 "The Gallup survey": W. H. Utian, 1994.

p. 97 "The beneficial effects of estrogen": J. C. Gallagher, 1993; R. Lindsay, 1991.

p. 97 "women who have a uterus and use supplementary estrogen": T. L. Bush, 1992.

p. 97 **"the use of adequate progestin"**: R. D. Gambrell, 1992.

p. 98 "the Progesterone Challenge Test": R. D. Gambrell, 1992.

p. 99 "testosterone can, in fact, be considered a 'weak estrogen' ": R. B. Greenblatt, 1987.

p. 99 " 'the presently available data support the concept' ": M. M. Gelfand, 1989.

p. 99 "A clinician with thirty years' experience": M. M. Gelfand, 1992.

p. 100 "Results of research designed to test the potential *benefit*": I. Karydas, 1987.

p. 100–101 "In fact, testosterone has been shown to exert": J. D. Wilson, 1980.

p. 101 "In 1995, statistics show": G. A. Colditz, 1995.

p. 101 "the three-year trial of estrogen and progesterone": Writing Group for the PEPI Trial, 1994.

p. 101 "As recently as June/July 1995": G. A. Colditz, 1995; J. L. Stanford, 1995.

p. 101 " 'More than fifty epidemiologic studies' ": American College of Obstetricians and Gynecologists Committee Opinion, 1994; D. Spicer, 1990.

p. 102 "A recent article by Jane Brody": J. Brody, 1994

CHAPTER EIGHT

p. 106 "A 1995 study": N. B. Watt, 1995.

p. 107 "an article by Dr. Greenblatt": R. B. Greenblatt, 1987.

p. 118 *"The British Medical Journal"*: H. Tunstall-Pedoe, 1997.

p. 118 "Rancho Bernardo Study": D. Kritz-Silverstein, 1997.

p. 119 "My paper, recently published": S. Rako, 1998.

৶ Bibliography ৹

American College of Obstetricians and Gynecologists Committee Opinion, "Estrogen Replacement Therapy in Women with Previously Treated Breast Cancer" (April 1994), no. 135.

Arafat, E. S., J. T. Hargrove, W. S. Maxson, D. M. Desiderio, A. Colston Wentz, and R. N. Andersen, "Sedative and Hypnotic Effects of Oral Administration of Micronized Progesterone May Be Mediated Through Its Metabolites," *American Journal of Obstetrics and Gynecology* 159, no. 5 (1988): 1203–09.

Bachmann, G. A., Estrogen-Androgen Therapy for Sexual and Emotional Well-Being," *The Female Patient* 18 (1993): 15–24.

Bancroft, J., "Hormones and Human Sexual Behaviour," *British Medical Bulletin* 37, no. 2 (1981): 153–58.

Bancroft, J., D. Sanders, D. Davidson, and P. Warner, "Mood, Sexuality, Hormones, and the Menstrual Cycle. III. Sexuality and the Role of Androgens," *Psychosomatic Medicine* 45, no. 6 (1983): 509–16.

Barrett-Connor, E, and K.-T. Khaw, "Absence of an Inverse Relation of Dehydroepiandrosterone Sulfate with Cardiovascular Mortality in Postmenopausal Women," *The New England Journal of Medicine* 317, no. 11 (1986): 711.

Barrett-Connor, E., K.-T. Khaw, and S. S. C. Yen, "A Prospective Study of Dehydroepiandrosterone Sulfate, Mortality, and Cardiovascular Disease," *The New England Journal of Medicine* 315, no. 24 (1986): 1519–24.

Brincat, M. A. Magos, J. W. W. Studd, L. D. Cardozo, T. O'Dowd, P. J. Wardle, and D. Cooper, "Subcutaneous Hormone Implants for the Control of Climacteric Symptoms," *The Lancet* (7 Jan. 1984): 16–18.

Brody, J. E., "Personal Health: Sex After Cancer: Planning Can Make a Major Difference," *New York Times,* 30 Nov. 1994: C11.

Burger, H. G., J. Hailes, M. Menelaus, J. Nelson, B. Hudson, and N.

Balazs, "The Management of Persistent Menopausal Symptoms with Oestradiol-Testosterone Implants: Clinical, Lipid and Hormonal Results," *Maturitas* 6 (1984): 351–58.

Bush, T. L., "Feminine Forever Revisited: Menopausal Hormone Therapy in the 1990s," *Journal of Women's Health* 1, no. 1 (1992): 1–4.

Campbell, B. C. and P. T. Ellison, "Menstrual Variation in Salivary Testosterone Among Regularly Cycling Women," *Hormone Research* 37 (1992): 132–36.

Cardozo, L. D., M. F. Gibb, S. M. Tuck, M. H. Thom, J. W. W. Studd, and D. J. Cooper, "The Effects of Subcutaneous Hormone Implants During the Climacteric," *Maturitas* 5 (1984): 177–84.

Chakravarti, S., W. P. Collins, J. R. Newton, D. H. Oram, and J. W. W. Studd, "Endocrine Changes and Symptomatology After Oophorectomy in Premenopausal Women," *British Journal of Obstetrics and Gynaecology* 84 (1977): 769–75.

Colditz, G. A., S. E. Hankinson, D. J. Hunter, W. C. Willett, J. E. Manson, M. J. Stampfer, C. Hennekens, B. Rosner and F. E. Speizer, "The Use of Estrogens and Progestins and the Risk of Breast Cancer in Postmenopausal Women," *The New England Journal of Medicine* 332, no. 24, (1995): 1589–1593.

Cole, E., Sex at Menopause: Each in Her Own Way," *Women and Therapy* 7 (1988): 159–68.

Cumming, D. C., R. W. Rebar, B. R. Hopper, and S. S. C. Yen, "Evidence for an Influence of the Ovary on Circulating Dehydroepiandrosterone Sulfate Levels," *Journal of Clinical Endocrinology and Metabolism* 54, no. 5 (1982): 1069–71.

Dabbs, Jr., J. M., "Salivary Testosterone Measurements: Reliability Across Hours, Days, and Weeks," *Psychology and Behavior* 48 (1990): 83–86.

———. "Salivary Testosterone Measurements: Collecting, Storing, and Mailing Saliva Samples," *Physiology and Behavior* 49 (1991): 815–17.

———. "Salivary Testosterone Measurements in Behavioral Studies." In *Saliva as a Diagnostic Fluid*, ed. D. Malamud and L. Tabak (*Annals of the New York Academy of Sciences:* 1993): 177–83.

Dabbs, Jr., J.M., and S. Mohammed, "Male and Female Salivary Testosterone Concentrations Before and After Sexual Activity," *Physiology and Behavior* 52 (1992): 195–97.

Dalton, K., *The Premenstrual Syndrome and Progesterone Therapy*. Chicago: Year Book Medical Publishers, Inc., 1977.

Daniel, S. A. J., and D. T. Armstrong, "Androgens in the Ovarian Microenvironment," *Seminars in Reproductive Endocrinology* 4, no. 2 (1986): 89–100.

Darj, E., O. Axelsson, K. Carlstrom, S. Nilsson, and B. von Schoultz, "Liver Metabolism During Treatment with Estradiol and Natural Progesterone," *Gynecological Endocrinology* 7, no. 2 (1993): 111–14.

Downey, J., "Infertility and the New Reproductive Technologies." In *Psy-*

chological Aspects of Women's Health Care, ed. C. E. Stewart and N. L. Stotland, American Psychiatric Press, Inc., (Washington, D.C.: 1993): 193–206.

Ebeling P., and V. A. Koivisto, "Physiological Importance of Dehydroepiandrosterone," *The Lancet* 343, no. 8911 (1994): 1479–81.

Elias, M., "Late-Life Love," *Harvard Health Letter* 18, no. 1 (Nov. 1992).

Fearnley, G. R., and R. Chakrabarti, "Increase of Blood Fibrinolytic Activity by Testosterone," *The Lancet* 2, no. 7247 (21 July, 1962): 128–132.

Feldman, H. A., I. Goldstein, D. G. Hatzichristou, R. J. Krane, and J. B. McKinlay, "Impotence and Its Medical and Psychosocial Correlates: Results of the Massachusetts Male Aging Study," *The Journal of Urology* 151 (1993): 54–61.

Finkelstein, J. S., A. Klibanski, R. M. Neer, S. H. Doppelt, D. I. Rosenthal, G. V. Segre, and W. F. Crowley, Jr., "Increases in Bone Density During Treatment of Men with Idiopathic Hypogonadotropic Hypogonadism," *Journal of Clinical Endocrinology and Metabolism* 69, no. 4 (1989): 776–82.

Finkelstein, J. S., R. M. Neer, B. M. K. Biller, J. D. Crawford, and A. Klibanski, "Osteopenia in Men with a History of Delayed Puberty," *The New England Journal of Medicine*, 326, no. 9, (1992): 600.

Freedman R. R., and J. H. Renner, "Natural/Alternative Therapies: Do They Have a Place in Treatment?" *Menopause Management* 3, no. 2 (1994): 24–27.

Friedrich, Jr., E. G., and P. S. Kalra, "Serum Levels of Sex Hormones in Vulvar Lichen Sclerosus, and the Effect of Topical Testosterone," *The New England Journal of Medicine* 310, no. 8 (1984): 488–91.

Furuyama, S., D. M. Mayes, and C. A. Nugent, "A Radioimmunoassay for Plasma Testosterone," *Steroids* 16, no. 4 (1970): 415–28.

Furuyama S., and C. A. Nugent, "A Radioimmunoassay for Plasma Progesterone," *Steroids* 17, no. 6 (1971): 663–74.

Gallagher, J. C., "Anti-resorptive Therapy in the Prevention of Osteoporosis," presented at the May 21, 1993, meeting of the North American Menopause Society and printed in the program book, *Menopause: The Background and Skills for Effective Therapy*, unnumbered.

Gambrell, R. D., "Complications of Estrogen Replacement Therapy." In *Hormone Replacement Therapy*, ed. D. P. Swartz (Baltimore: Williams & Wilkins, 1992): 191–219.

Geist, S. H., "Androgen Therapy in the Human Female," *Journal of Clinical Endocrinology* 1, no. 2 (1941): 154–61.

Geist, S. H., and U. J. Salmon, "Androgen Therapy in Gynecology," *Journal of the American Medical Association* 117, no. 26 (1941): 2207–13.

Gelfand, M. M., "Estrogen-Androgen Hormone Replacement Therapy." In *Hormone Replacement Therapy*, ed. D. P. Swartz (Baltimore: Williams & Wilkins, 1992): 221–34.

Gelfand, M. M., A. Ferenczy, and C. Bergeron, "Endometrial Response to

Estrogen-Androgen Stimulation." In *Menopause: Evaluation, Treatment, and Health Concerns,* ed. C. B. Hammond and F. P. Haseltine (New York: Alan R. Liss, Inc., 1989): 29–40.

George, A., and M. Sandler, "Endocrine and Biochemical Studies in Puerperal Mental Disorders." In *Motherhood and Mental Illness,* vol. 2 *Causes and Consequences,* ed. R. Kumar and I. F. Brockington (London: Wright, 1988): 78–112.

Greenblatt, R. B., "Androgenic Therapy in Women," *Journal of Clinical Endocrinology* 2, (1942): 665–66.

———. "Hormone Factors in Libido," *Journal of Clinical Endocrinology* 3, no. 5 (1943): 305–06.

———. "Syndrome of Nocturnal Frequency Alleviated by Testosterone Propionate," *Journal of Clinical Endocrinology* 2, no. 5 (1942): 321–24.

———. "The Use of Androgens in the Menopause and Other Gynecic Disorders," *Obstetrics and Gynecology Clinics of North America* 14, no. 1 (1987): 251–68.

Greenblatt, R. B., W. E. Barfield, J. F. Garner, G. L. Calk, and J. P. Harrod, Jr., "Evaluation of an Estrogen, Androgen, Estrogen-Androgen Combination, and a Placebo in the Treatment of the Menopause," *Journal of Clinical Endocrinology* 2, no. 11 (1950): 1547–58.

Greenblatt, R. B., J. S. Chaddha, A. Z. Teran, and C. H. Nezhat, "Aphrodisiacs." In *Psychopharmacology: Recent Advances and Future Prospects,* ed. S. D. Iversom (New York: Oxford University Press, Inc., 1985): 289–302.

Greenblatt, R. B., M. L. Colle, and V. B. Mahesh, "Ovarian and Adrenal Steroid Production in the Postmenopausal Woman," *Journal of Obstetrics and Gynecology* 47, no. 4 (1976): 383–87.

Greer, G., *The Change.* New York: Random House, 1992.

Hallstrom, T., "Sexuality in the Climacteric," *Clinics in Obstetrics and Gynaecology* 4, no. 1 (1977): 227–39.

Hargrove, J. T., W. S. Maxson, and A. Colston Wentz, "Absorption of Oral Progesterone Is Influenced by Vehicle and Particle Size," *American Journal of Obstetrics and Gynecology* 161, no. 4 (1989): 948–51.

Hargrove, J. T., W. S. Maxson, A. Colston Wentz, and L. S. Burnett, "Menopausal Hormone Replacement Therapy with Continuous Daily Oral Micronized Estradiol and Progesterone," *Obstetrics and Gynecology* 73, no. 4 (1989): 606–12.

Haseltine, F. P., G. P. Redmond, A. Colston Wentz, and R. A. Wild, "Introduction," *The American Journal of Medicine (Proceedings of a Symposium: An NICHD Conference; Androgens and Women's Health)* 98 (1A) (1995): 1S.

Henrich, J. B., "The Postmenopausal Estrogen/Breast Cancer Controversy," *Journal of the American Medical Association* 268, no. 14 (1992): 1900–02.

Hufnagel. V., *No More Hysterectomies*. New York and Scarborough, Ontario: New American Library, 1988.

Hulka, B. S., E. T. Liu, and R. A. Lininger, "Steroid Hormones and Risk of Breast Cancer," *Cancer* 74, no. 3 (1993): 1111–24.

Hutchinson, K. A., "Androgens and Sexuality," *The American Journal of Medicine (Proceedings of a Symposium: An NICHD Conference; Androgens and Women's Health)* 98 (1A) (1995): 111S–119S.

Jaffe, M. D., "Effect of Testosterone Cypionate on Postexercise ST Segment Depression," *British Heart Journal* 39 (1977): 1217–22.

Jarrahi-Zadeh, A., F. J. Kane, R. L. Van de Castle, P. A. Lachenbruch, and J. A. Ewing, "Emotional and Cognitive Changes in Pregnancy and Early Puerperium," *British Journal of Psychiatry* 115 (1969): 797–805.

Jensvold, M. F., "Psychiatric Aspects of the Menstrual Cycle." In *Motherhood and Mental Illness*, vol. 2 *Causes and Consequences*, ed. R. Kumar and I. F. Brockington (London: Wright, 1988): 165–92.

Judd, H. L., G. E. Judd, W. E. Lucas, and S. S. C. Yen, "Endocrine Function of the Postmenopausal Ovary: Concentration of Androgens and Estrogens in Ovarian and Peripheral Vein Blood," *Journal of Clinical Endocrinology and Metabolism* 39, no. 6 (1974): 1020–24.

Kaplan, H. S., "A Neglected Issue: The Sexual Side Effects of Current Treatments for Breast Cancer," *Journal of Sex and Marital Therapy* 18, no. 1 (1992): 3–19.

Kaplan, H. S., and T. Owett, "The Female Androgen Deficiency Syndrome," *Journal of Sex and Marital Therapy* 19, no. 1 (1992): 3–24.

Kaptchuk, T. J., *The Web That Has No Weaver*. Chicago: Contemporary Books, Inc., 1984.

Karydas, I., I. S. Fentiman, D. Tong, R. D. Bulbrook, and J. L. Hayward, "Adjuvant Androgen Treatment of Operable Breast Cancer—a 20 Year Analysis," *European Journal of Surgical Oncology* 13 (1987): 113–17.

Klaiber, E. L., D. M. Broverman, C. I. Haffajee, J. S. Hochman and J. E. Dalen, "Serum Estrogen Levels in Men with Acute Myocardial Infarction," *The American Journal of Medicine* 73, (1982): 872–881.

Kritz-Silverstein, D., E. Barret-Connor, and D. L. Wingard. "Hysterectomy, Oophorectomy, and Heart Disease Risk Factors in Older Women." *American Journal of Public Health* 87, no. 4 (1997): 676–80.

Kronenberg, F., "Alternative Therapies: New Opportunities for Menopause Research" (editorial), *Menopause* 2, no. 1 (1995): 1–2.

Legro, R. S., "The Genetics of Polycystic Ovary Syndrome," *The American Journal of Medicine (Proceedings of a Symposium: An NICHD Conference; Androgens and Women's Health)* 98 (1A) (1995): 9S–16S.

Lesser, M. A., "Testosterone Propionate Therapy in One Hundred Cases of Angina Pectoris," *The Journal of Clinical Endocrinology* 6, no. 7 (1946): 549–57.

Lindsay, R., and F. Cosman, "The Risk of Osteoporosis in Aging Women,"

The Menopause and Hormonal Replacement Therapy, ed. R. Sitruk-Ware and W. H. Utian, (New York: Marcel Dekker, Inc., 1991): 47–72.

Lobo, R. A., "Estrogens and Heart Disease" (paper presented at the May 21, 1993, meeting of the North American Menopause Society and printed in its program book, *Menopause: The Background and Skills for Effective Therapy,* unnumbered).

Longcope, C., "Adrenal and Gonadal Androgen Secretion in Normal Females," *Clinics in Endocrinology and Metabolism* 15 no. 2 (1986): 213–28.

Longcope, C., R. Hunter, and C. Franz, "Steroid Secretion by the Postmenopausal Ovary," *American Journal of Obstetrics and Gynecology* 138 (1980): 564–68.

Love, R. R., "Hormone Treatment in Women With Excellent-Prognosis Breast Cancer," *Oncology* (Williston Park) 4, no. 12 (1990): 59–62.

McBride, G., *The Harvard Health Letter: A Special Report: Postmenopausal Hormone-Replacement Therapy* (1993).

McCoy, N. L., "The Menopause and Sexuality," *The Menopause and Hormone Replacement Therapy,* (New York: Marcel Dekker, Inc.), R. Sitruk-Ware and W. U. Utian, eds., (1991): 73–100.

McCoy, N. L., and J. M. Davidson, "A Longitudinal Study of the Effects of Menopause on Sexuality," *Maturitas* 7 (1985): 203–10.

McEwen, B. S., "Gonadal Hormone Receptors in Developing and Adult Brain: Relationship to the Regulatory Phenotype." In *Fetal Neuroendocrinology,* ed. F. Ellendorff, P. Gluckman, and N. Parvizi (Ithaca, N.Y.: Perinatology Press, 1984): 149–159.

———. "Sex Differences in the Brain." In *Women and Men: New Perspectives in Gender Differences,* ed. C. Nadelson and M. Notman (Washington, D.C.: American Psychiatric Press, Inc., 1991): 35–41.

McKinlay, J. B., "The Prevalence of Impotence and Its Medical and Psychosocial Correlates," *Journal of the American Medical Association* 270 (1993): 83–90.

McKinlay, J. B., and H. A. Feldman, "Age-Related Variation in Sexual Activity and Interest in Normal Men: Results from the Massachusetts Male Aging Study." In *Sexuality Across the Life Course: Proceedings of the MacArthur Foundation Research Network on Successful Mid-Life Development,* ed. Alice S. Rossi (Chicago: The University of Chicago Press, 1994): 261–85.

McKinlay, J. B., C. Longcope, and A. Gray, "The Questionable Physiologic and Epidemiologic Basis for a Male Climacteric Syndrome: Preliminary Results from the Massachusetts Male Aging Study," *Maturitas* 11 (1989): 103–15.

McKinlay, J. B., S. M. McKinlay, and D. Brambilla, "The Relative Contributions of Endocrine Changes and Social Circumstances to Depression in Mid-Aged Women," *Journal of Health and Social Behavior* 28 (1987): 345–63.

Miller, L. J., "Psychiatric Disorders During Pregnancy." In *Psychological Aspects of Women's Health Care,* ed. C. E. Stewart and N. L. Stotland (Washington, D.C.: American Psychiatric Press, Inc., 1993): 55–70.

Money, J., "Components of Eroticism in Man: 1. The Hormones in Relation to Sexual Morphology and Sexual Desire," *Journal of Nervous and Mental Diseases* 132 (1961): 239–48.

Morales, A. J., J. J. Nolan, J. C. Nelson, and S. S. C. Yen, "Effects of Replacement Dose of Dehydroepiandrosterone in Men and Women of Advancing Age," *Journal of Clinical Endocrinology and Metabolism* 78, no. 6 (1994): 1360–67.

Orentreich, N., J. L. Brind, R. L. Rizer, and J. H. Vogelman, "Age Changes and Sex Differences in Serum Dehydroepiandrosterone Sulfate Concentrations Throughout Adulthood," *Journal of Clinical Endocrinology and Metabolism* 59, no. 3 (1984): 551–55.

Persky, H., N. Charney, H. I. Leif, C. P. O'Brien, W. R. Miller, and D. Strauss, "The Relationship of Plasma Estradiol Level to Sexual Behavior in Young Women," *Psychosomatic Medicine* 40, no. 7 (1978): 523–35.

Persky, H., L. Dreisbach, W. R. Miller, C. P. O'Brien, M. A. Khan, H. I. Lief, N. Charney, and D. Strauss, "The Relation of Plasma Androgen Levels to Sexual Behaviors and Attitudes of Women," *Psychosomatic Medicine* 44, no. 4 (1982): 305–19.

Persky, H., H. I. Leif, D. Strauss, W. R. Miller, and C. P. O'Brien, "Plasma Testosterone Level and Sexual Behavior in Couples," *Archives of Sexual Behavior* 7, no. 3 (1978): 157–73.

Pfeiffer, E., A. Verwoerdt, and G. C. Davis, "Sexual Behavior in Middle Life," *American Journal of Psychiatry* 128, no. 10 (1972): 1262–68.

Phillips, G. B., B. H. Pinkernell, and T.-Y. Jing, "The Association of Hypotestosteronemia With Coronary Artery Disease in Men," *Arteriosclerosis and Thrombosis* 14, no. 5, (1994): 701.

Poulin, R., D. Baker, and F. Labrie, "Androgens Inhibit Basal and Estrogen-Induced Cell Proliferation in the ZR-75-1 Human Breast Cancer Cell Line," *Breast Cancer Research and Treatment* 12 (1988): 213–25.

Prior, J. C., Y. M. Vigna, M. T. Schechter, and A. E. Burgess, "Spinal Bone Loss and Ovulatory Disturbances," *The New England Journal of Medicine* 323, no. 18 (1990): 1221–27.

Rako, S., "Testosterone Deficiency: A Key Factor in the Increased Cardiovascular Risk to Women Following Hysterectomy or with Natural Aging?" *Journal of Women's Health* 7, no. 7 (1998): 825–29.

Ravn, S. H., J. Rosenberg, and E. Bostofte, "Postmenopausal Hormone Replacement Therapy—Clinical Implications," *European Journal of Obstetrics, Gynecology, and Reproductive Biology* 53, no. 2 (1994): 81–93.

Regelson, W., R. Loria, and M. Kalimi, "Dehydroepiandrosterone (DHEA)—the 'Mother Steroid,' " *Annals of the New York Academy of Sciences* 719 (1994): 553.

Rittmaster, R. S., "Clinical Relevance of Testosterone and Dihydrotestosterone Metabolism in Women," *The American Journal of Medicine (Proceedings of a Symposium: An NICHD Conference: Androgens and Women's Health)* 98 (1A) (1995): 17S–26S.

Rose, R. M., "The Psychological Effects of Androgens and Estrogens—A Review." In *Psychiatric Complications of Medical Drugs,* ed. R. Shader (New York: Raven Press, 1972): 251–93.

Rosenfield, R. L., and D. Deplewski, "Role of Androgens in the Developmental Biology of the Pilosebaceous Unit," *The American Journal of Medicine (Proceedings of a Symposium: An NICHD Conference: Androgens and Women's Health)* 98 (1A) (1995): 805–885.

Salmon, U. J., and S. H. Geist, "Effect of Androgens upon Libido in Women," *Journal of Clinical Endocrinology* 3 (1943): 235–38.

Sands, R., and J. Studd, "Exogenous Androgens in Postmenopausal Women," *The American Journal of Medicine (Proceedings of a Symposium: An NICHD Conference: Androgens and Women's Health)* 98 (1A) (1995): 76S–79S.

Sherwin, B. B., "Affective Changes with Estrogen and Androgen Replacement Therapy in Surgically Menopausal Women," *Journal of Affective Disorders* 14 (1988): 177–87.

———. "Menopause: Myths and Realities." In *Psychological Aspects of Women's Health Care,* ed. C. E. Stewart and N. L. Stotland (Washington, D.C.: American Psychiatric Press, Inc., 1993): 227–48.

Sherwin, B. B., and M. M. Gelfand, "Differential Symptom Response to Parenteral Estrogen and/or Androgen Administration in the Surgical Menopause," *American Journal of Obstetrics and Gynecology* 151, no. 2 (1985): 153–60.

———. "Sex Steroids and Affect in the Surgical Menopause: A Double-Blind, Cross-Over Study," *Psychoneuroendocrinology* 10, no. 3 (1985): 325–35.

———. "The Role of Androgen in the Maintenance of Sexual Functioning in Oophorectomized Women," *Psychosomatic Medicine* 49, no. 4 (1987): 397–409.

Sherwin, B. B., M. M. Gelfand, and W. Brender, "Androgen Enhances Sexual Motivation in Females: A Prospective, Crossover Study of Sex Steroid Administration in the Surgical Menopause," *Psychosomatic Medicine* 47, no. 4 (1985): 339–51.

Sherwin, B. B., M. M. Gelfand, R. Schucher, and J. Gabor, "Postmenopausal Estrogen and Androgen Replacement and Lipoprotein Lipid Concentrations," *American Journal of Obstetrics and Gynecology* 156, no. 2 (1987): 414–19.

Sitruk-Ware R., and W. Utian, eds. *The Menopause and Hormonal Replacement Therapy: Facts and Controversies.* New York: Marcel Dekker, Inc., 1991.

Spicer, D., M. C. Pike, and B. E. Henderson, "The Question of Estrogen Replacement Therapy in Patients With a Prior Diagnosis of Breast Cancer," *Oncology* (Williston Park) 4, no. 12 (1990): 49–54.

Stanford, J. L., N. S. Weiss, L. F. Voigt, J. R. Daling, L. A. Habel, and M. A. Rossing, "Combined Estrogen and Progestin Hormone Replacement Therapy in Relation to Risk of Breast Cancer in Middle Aged Women," *Journal of the American Medical Association,* 274, no. 2, (1995): 137.

Stein, I. F., and M. L. Leventhal, "Amenorrhea Associated with Bilateral Polycystic Ovaries," *American Journal of Obstetrics and Gynecology* 29 (1935): 181–91.

Stewart, D. E., and N. L. Stotland, "The Interface Between Psychiatry and Obstetrics and Gynecology: An Introduction." In *Psychological Aspects of Women's Health Care,* ed. D. E. Stewart and N. L. Stotland (Washington, D.C.: American Psychiatric Press, Inc., 1993): 1–11.

Studd, J. W. W., W. P. Collins, S. Chakravarti, J. R. Newton, D. Oram, and A. Parsons, "Oestradiol and Testosterone Implants in the Treatment of Psychosexual Problems in the Post-Menopausal Woman," *British Journal of Obstetrics and Gynecology* 84 (1977): 314–16.

Tainter, M. L., A. Arnold, A. L. Beyler, G. O. Potts, and C. H. Roth, "Anabolic Steroids in the Management of the Diabetic Patient," *New York State Journal of Medicine"* (April 15, 1964): 1001–09.

Tenover, J. S., "Effects of Testosterone Supplementation in the Aging Male," *Journal of Clinical Endocrinology and Metabolism* 75, no. 4 (1992): 1092–98.

Tufts University Diet and Nutrition Letter, "Scientists Spotlight Phytoestrogens for Better Health," 12, no. 12 (1995).

Tunstall-Pedoe, H., M. Woodward, R. Tavendale, R. A'Brook, and M. K. McCluskey. "Comparison of the Prediction by 27 Different Factors of Coronary Heart Disease and Death in Men and Women of the Scottish Heart Health Study: Cohort Study." *The British Medical Journal* 315 (1997): 722–29.

Utian, W. H., and I. Schiff, "NAMS-Gallup Survey on Women's Knowledge, Information Sources, and Attitudes to Menopause and Hormone Replacement Therapy," *Menopause* 1, no. 1 (1994): 39–59.

Verhaar, H. J., C. A. Damen, S. A. Duursma, and B. A. Scheven, "A Comparison of the Action of Progestins and Estrogen on the Growth and Differentiation of Normal Adult Human Osteoblast-like Cells in Vitro," *Bone* 15, no. 3 (1994): 307–11.

Villareal, D. T., and J. E. Morley, "Trophic Factors in Aging: Should Older People Receive Hormonal Replacement Therapy?" *Drugs and Aging* 4, no. 6 (1994): 492–509.

Vittek, J., D. G. L'Hommedieu, G. G. Gordon, S. C. Rappaport, and A. L. Southren, "Direct Radioimmunoassay (RAI) of Salivary Testosterone, Correlation with Free and Total Serum Testosterone," *Life Sciences* 37 (1985): 711–16.

Watts, N. B., M. Notelovitz, M. C. Timmons, W. A. Addison, B. Wiita, and L. J. Downey. "Comparison of Oral Estrogens Plus Androgen on Bone Mineral Density, Menopausal Symptoms, and Lipid-lipoprotein profiles in Surgical Menopause." *Obstetrics and Gynecology* 85, no. 4 (1995): 529–37.

Waxenberg, S. E., M. G. Drellich, and A. M. Sutherland, "The Role of Hormones in Human Behavior. I. Changes in Female Sexuality After Adrenalectomy," *Journal of Clinical Endocrinology* 19 (1959): 193–202.

Waxenberg, S. E., J. A. Finkbeiner, M. G. Drellich, and A. M. Sutherland, "The Role of Hormones in Human Behavior. II. Changes in Sexual Behavior in Relation to Vaginal Smears of Breast-Cancer Patients After Oophorectomy and Adrenalectomy," *Psychosomatic Medicine* 22, no. 6 (1960): 435–42.

Weed. S. S., *Menopausal Years.* Woodstock, N.Y.: Ash Tree Publishing, 1992.

Wilson, J. D., J. Aiman, and P. C. MacDonald, "The Pathogenesis of Gynecomastia," *Advances in Internal Medicine* 25, no. 1, (1980): 1.

Wise, P. M., N. G. Weiland, K. Scarbrough, M. A. Sortino, I. R. Cohen, and G. H. Larson, "Changing Hypothalamopituitary Function: Its Role in Aging of the Female Reproductive System," *Hormone Research* 31 (1989): 39–44.

Wright, A. J., "Testosterone Pellet Implant Therapy for Lichen Sclerosus," *Missouri Medicine* 90, no. 11 (1993): 711–13.

Writing Group for the PEPI Trial, "Effects of Estrogen or Estrogen/Progestin Regimens on Heart Disease Risk Factors in Postmenopausal Women: The Postmenopausal Estrogen/Progestin Interventions (PEPI) Trial," *The Journal of the American Medical Association* 273, no. 3 (1994): 199–208.

Yamaguchi, A., T. Ichimura, and T. Yamabe, "The Measurement of Plasma-Free Testosterone in Normal Menstrual Females, Pregnant Females, Post Menopausal Females and Vulvar Dystrophy," *Folia Endocrinologica Japonica* 64, no. 6 (1988): 482–88.

Yen, S. S. C., "Chronic Anovulation Caused by Peripheral Endocrine Disorders," *Reproductive Endocrinology* (W. B. Saunders), S. S. C. Yen and R. B. Jaffe, eds. (1991): 576–630.

Yen, S. S. C., and R. B. Jaffe eds. *Reproductive Endocrinology.* Philadelphia: W. B. Saunders Company, 1991.

Young, R. L., "Androgens in Postmenopausal Therapy?" *Menopause Management* 2, no. 5 (1993): 21–24.

ᨏ Index ᨏ

↬ About the Author ↫

SUSAN RAKO, M.D., has been a psychiatrist in private practice in the Boston area for nearly thirty years. She both trained and taught at Harvard Medical School's Massachusetts Mental Health Center, a teaching hospital in the Department of Psychiatry. She attended Wellesley College through her junior year and earned her M.D. from Albert Einstein College of Medicine in New York, where she was one of five women in a class of one hundred. Her graduation in 1966 was attended by her daughter, Jennifer, then two and a half years old.

With developed interests in writing and film, Dr. Rako earned a master's degree in film from Boston University's College of Communication in 1988, just before her hormones crashed. The search and discovery that followed became the project that generated this book.

"It was not my initial intention to teach about testosterone deficiency and menopause," she says, "but I know that the knowledge I have gained must be more widely shared."

Dr. Rako is at work on a collection of stories and lessons from a life.